The MAX
Muscle Plan

The MAX Muscle Plan

Brad Schoenfeld

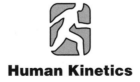

Human Kinetics

Library of Congress Cataloging-in-Publication Data

Schoenfeld, Brad, 1962-
  The max muscle plan / Brad Schoenfeld.
      p. cm.
  Includes bibliographical references.
  1. Bodybuilding. 2. Muscle strength. I. Title.
  GV546.5.S36 2012
  613.7'13--dc23

                            2012018675

ISBN-10: 1-4504-2387-6 (print)
ISBN-13: 978-1-4504-2387-8 (print)

Acquisitions Editor: Justin Klug; **Developmental Editor:** Carla Zych; **Assistant Editor:** Claire Marty; **Copyeditor:** Amanda M. Eastin-Allen; **Graphic Designer:** Joe Buck; **Cover Designer:** Keith Blomberg; **Photographs (cover and interior):** Neil Bernstein and Doug Fink; **Visual Production Assistant:** Joyce Brumfield; **Photo Production Manager:** Jason Allen; **Printer:** United Graphics

We thank Adrenaline Gym in Peekskill, NY, for assistance in providing the location for the photo shoot for this book.

Human Kinetics books are available at special discounts for bulk purchase. Special editions or book excerpts can also be created to specification. For details, contact the Special Sales Manager at Human Kinetics.

Printed in the United States of America   10 9 8 7 6 5 4 3 2 1

The paper in this book is certified under a sustainable forestry program.

Human Kinetics
Website: www.HumanKinetics.com

United States: Human Kinetics
P.O. Box 5076
Champaign, IL 61825-5076
800-747-4457
e-mail: humank@hkusa.com

Canada: Human Kinetics
475 Devonshire Road Unit 100
Windsor, ON N8Y 2L5
800-465-7301 (in Canada only)
e-mail: info@hkcanada.com

Europe: Human Kinetics
107 Bradford Road
Stanningley
Leeds LS28 6AT, United Kingdom
+44 (0) 113 255 5665
e-mail: hk@hkeurope.com

Australia: Human Kinetics
57A Price Avenue
Lower Mitcham, South Australia 5062
08 8372 0999
e-mail: info@hkaustralia.com

New Zealand: Human Kinetics
P.O. Box 80
Torrens Park, South Australia 5062
0800 222 062
e-mail: info@hknewzealand.com

E5646

This book is humbly dedicated to all the researchers who have expanded my knowledge of exercise science and thus provided the underlying basis for this book.

Contents

Exercise Finder

Exercise	Primary muscles worked	Other muscles worked	Single joint or multijoint	Page #
CHAPTER 3 EXERCISES FOR THE BACK, CHEST, AND ABDOMEN				
Back				
Dumbbell pullover	lats, sternal pectorals		Single	26
Dumbbell one-arm row	inner-back muscles, back		Multi	27
T-bar row	back muscles		Multi	28
Barbell reverse-grip bent row	back muscles		Multi	29
Barbell overhand bent row	back muscles		Multi	30
Machine close-grip seated row	rhomboids, middle traps, back muscles		Multi	31
Machine wide-grip seated row	posterior deltoid, back muscles		Multi	32
Cable seated row	rhomboids, middle traps, back muscles		Multi	33
Cable wide-grip seated row	posterior deltoid, back muscles		Multi	34
Cable one-arm standing low row	back muscles		Multi	35
Chin-up	back muscles	biceps	Multi	36
Pull-up	back muscles		Multi	37
Lat pull-down	lats, back muscles		Multi	38
Neutral-grip lat pull-down	back muscles		Multi	39
Reverse-grip lat pull-down	back muscles		Multi	40
Cable straight-arm lat pull-down	lats, back muscles		Single	41
Cross cable lat pull-down	lats, back muscles		Multi	42
Chest				
Dumbbell incline press	upper chest, pectorals, triceps, front delts		Multi	43
Dumbbell decline press	lower aspect of the pectorals, triceps		Multi	44
Dumbbell chest press	sternal pectorals		Multi	45
Barbell incline press	upper chest, pectorals, triceps, front delts		Multi	46
Barbell chest press	sternal pectorals, triceps, front delts		Multi	47

Exercise	Primary muscles worked	Other muscles worked	Single joint or multijoint	Page #
Chest (*continued*)				
Barbell decline press	lower chest, pectorals, triceps, front delts		Multi	48
Machine incline press	upper pectorals	shoulders, triceps	Multi	49
Machine chest press	sternal pectorals		Multi	50
Dumbbell flat fly	sternal pectorals		Single	51
Dumbbell incline fly	upper fibers of the pectorals		Single	52
Pec deck fly	chest muscles		Single	53
Cable fly	sternal pectorals		Single	54
Chest dip	lower pectorals		Multi	55
Abdomen				
Crunch	upper abdominal region		Multi	56
Reverse crunch	lower abdominal region		Multi	57
Bicycle crunch	abs		Multi	58
Roman chair side crunch	obliques		Multi	59
Stability ball abdominal crunch	abs		Multi	60
Cable rope kneeling crunch	upper portion of the abs		Multi	61
Cable rope kneeling twisting crunch	abs, obliques		Multi	62
Toe touch	upper abdominal region		Multi	63
Plank	core		N/A	64
Side bridge	core		N/A	65
Hanging knee raise	abs		Multi	66
Russian twist	obliques		Multi	67
Dumbbell side bend	obliques		Multi	68
Cable side bend	obliques		Multi	69
Cable wood chop	obliques		Multi	70
Barbell rollout	abs		Multi	71

(continued)

Exercise	Primary muscles worked	Other muscles worked	Single joint or multijoint	Page #
CHAPTER 4 EXERCISES FOR THE SHOULDERS AND ARMS				
Shoulders				
Arnold press	deltoids	upper trapezius, triceps	Multi	74
Military press	front delts, shoulders	upper trapezius, triceps	Multi	75
Dumbbell shoulder press	front delts, deltoids	upper trapezius, triceps	Multi	76
Machine shoulder press	front delts, deltoids	upper trapezius, triceps	Multi	77
Dumbbell lateral raise	middle delts		Single	78
Machine lateral raise	middle delts		Single	79
Cable lateral raise	middle delts		Single	80
Dumbbell bent reverse fly	posterior deltoid		Single	81
Machine rear delt fly	posterior deltoid		Single	82
Cable reverse fly	posterior deltoid		Single	83
Cable kneeling reverse fly	posterior deltoid		Single	84
Barbell upright row	middle delts	biceps	Multi	85
Cable upright row	middle delts	biceps	Multi	86
Biceps				
Dumbbell standing biceps curl	biceps		Single	87
Dumbbell incline biceps curl	long head, biceps		Single	88
Dumbbell facedown incline curl	short head, biceps		Single	89
Dumbbell preacher curl	short head, biceps		Single	90
Barbell preacher curl	short head, biceps		Single	91
Machine preacher curl	short head, biceps		Single	92
Concentration curl	short head, biceps		Single	93
Dumbbell standing hammer curl	brachialis, upper arms		Single	94
Barbell curl	biceps		Single	95
Barbell drag curl	long head, biceps		Single	96
Cable rope hammer curl	brachialis, upper arms		Single	97
Cable curl	biceps		Single	98
Cable one-arm curl	biceps		Single	99

Exercise	Primary muscles worked	Other muscles worked	Single joint or multijoint	Page #
Triceps				
Dumbbell overhead triceps extension	long head, triceps		Single	100
Cable rope overhead triceps extension	long head, triceps		Single	101
Nosebreaker	triceps		Single	102
Machine nosebreaker	triceps		Single	103
Dumbbell triceps kickback	middle and lateral heads, triceps		Single	104
Cable triceps kickback	middle and lateral heads, triceps		Single	105
Bench press	pecs, triceps		Single	106
Cable triceps press-down	middle and lateral heads, triceps		Single	107
Triceps dip	triceps		Single	108
Machine triceps dip	triceps		Single	109
CHAPTER 5 EXERCISES FOR THE LOWER BODY				
Multijoint exercises				
Walking lunge	quads, glutes	hamstrings	Multi	112
Barbell lunge	quads, glutes	hamstrings	Multi	113
Dumbbell lunge	quads, glutes	hamstrings	Multi	114
Dumbbell reverse lunge	quads, glutes	hamstrings	Multi	115
Dumbbell side lunge	adductors, all lower body		Multi	116
Dumbbell step-up	quads, glutes	hamstrings	Multi	117
Barbell front squat	frontal thighs, quads, glutes	hamstrings	Multi	118
Barbell back squat	quads, glutes	hamstrings	Multi	119
Barbell split squat	quads, glutes	hamstrings	Multi	120
Bulgarian squat	quads, glutes	hamstrings	Multi	121
Leg press	quads, glutes	hamstrings	Multi	122
Deadlift	all lower body	upper-body muscles	Multi	123
Single-joint exercises				
Good morning	glutes, hamstrings		Single	124
Sissy squat	rectus femoris, quads		Single	125
Barbell stiff-legged deadlift	glutes, hamstrings		Single	126
Dumbbell stiff-legged deadlift	glutes, hamstrings		Single	127

(continued)

Exercise Finder *(continued)*

Exercise	Primary muscles worked	Other muscles worked	Single joint or multijoint	Page #
Single-joint exercises *(continued)*				
Cable glute kickback	gluteus maximus, glutes, hamstrings		Single	128
Hyperextension	glutes, hamstrings		Single	129
Reverse hyperextension	glutes, hamstrings		Single	130
Leg extension	quads		Single	131
One-leg extension	quads		Single	132
Lying leg curl	hamstrings		Single	133
Machine kneeling leg curl	hamstrings		Single	134
Machine seated leg curl	hamstrings		Single	135
Toe press	calf muscles		Single	136
Machine seated calf raise	soleus, calf muscles		Single	137
Machine standing calf raise	calf muscles		Single	138

Foreword

Exercise science is a relatively young field in the pantheon of science. When exercise science first entered the fray, it was somewhat dismissed as unimportant and even vain. Over the past quarter of a century, however, the world has come to recognize the importance of exercise in promoting health, well-being, and longevity. With this recognition has come a plethora of new information regarding training protocols. This is both a good thing and a bad thing. Valid research on proper training protocols has expanded by leaps and bounds over the past few decades; however, pseudoscience and outright untruthful claims have expanded at an equal pace. Unfortunately, where money can be made, scam artists will prop up gimmicks in order to make a quick buck. This has led to legions of books, DVDs, and websites promoting ineffective training protocols as the simple solution. After all, who doesn't want to get a ripped six-pack by working out one minute per day, two days per year? Most of us would love the idea of working out very little and getting great results. Unfortunately, progress requires hard work. Many books bend the truth in order to sell a magic formula that doesn't involve hard work. *The MAX Muscle Plan* is not one of those books.

In *The MAX Muscle Plan*, Brad Schoenfeld breaks down the science behind training and periodization and explains how to properly implement these components. He dissects complex research and provides recommendations that can be implemented by the average Joe who doesn't have a PhD in exercise physiology. Brad helps you better understand how to organize your training and how to properly implement workout protocols in order to maximize their effectiveness and meet your goals. This book gives you the path to success in your weight-training goals; it is up to you to walk that path. There are no easy ways to the finish line, and there are no quick fixes. It will take nothing short of hard work and dedication to reach your weight-training and physique goals, but this book gives you the road map that will lead you toward them.

Best of luck on your journey.
Layne Norton, PhD

Acknowledgments

This book was many years in the making and there are a number of people I would like to thank for helping see it to fruition.

To my brother, Glenn Schoenfeld: Thank you, first off, for doing such an awesome job as one of the demonstration models and enduring multiple takes of exercise after exercise, but more importantly, for facilitating my entrance into the fitness field and helping me when I needed it most. I would not be where I am today without your support and guidance!

To Carlos and John of Adrenaline Gym in Peekskill, New York: I can't thank you enough for making your awesome training facility available for the photo shoot. You have a gem of a gym; it's one of the few hard-core facilities left!

To demonstration models Michael Vasquez, Kenneth Figueroa, Rich Berta, Rich Herrera: Many thanks for putting up with the grueling demands of the photo shoot and performing a seemingly endless number of takes for each exercise without an ounce of complaint. You guys are total pros!

To Doug Fink and Neil Bernstein: It was great to work with you guys again on another photo shoot. You always do an excellent job and this time you went above and beyond.

To the editorial staff at Human Kinetics and, in particular, Jason Muzinic, Justin Klug, and Carla Zych: You helped bring my vision to life, and I couldn't be happier with the final product. Your efforts are greatly appreciated.

To Bret Contreras: Many thanks for your keen eye in reviewing the training chapters. You are a great friend and colleague!

To Alan Aragon: I really appreciate your thorough and insightful review of the nutrition chapter. You are a credit to the industry, and I am proud to call you a friend!

To Layne Norton: I'm honored that you agreed to write the foreword to my book. You are a role model to many, and you epitomize the essence of bodybuilding. Huge thanks!

Finally, to my parents: You instilled the importance of the scientific method in me from an early age, and it has shaped who I am. I love you both always. Rest in peace, Dad.

Introduction

If you're reading this book, it's safe to bet that you want to achieve a better body. If so, great! You've come to the right source.

Why choose *The MAX Muscle Plan* rather than one of the hundreds of other books promising a direct route to physique heaven? Fair question. Truth be told, you can gain muscle by following pretty much any resistance training program—at least in the early phases of training. Simply challenge your body beyond its present capacity with reasonably heavy weights, and your muscles will adapt by getting bigger. Unfortunately, such an approach will take you only so far. Without a well-devised plan of action, you'll soon reach a plateau and results will come crashing to a halt.

Many people figure the best way to keep packing on muscle is by emulating the training methods of their favorite bodybuilders. They subscribe to various bodybuilding magazines and piece together routines consisting of the "ultimate Mr. Olympia arm workout" and "Mr. America's secrets to massive thighs." On the surface, such an approach seems perfectly logical. After all, a pro bodybuilder must know a thing or two about how to get big, right?

Fact is, bodybuilders often achieve their superhuman physiques through a combination of great genetics and a whole lot of chemical enhancement. So unless your genetics are similar to those of the pros (highly unlikely) and you are willing to take massive doses of anabolic agents and pharmaceuticals (highly risky), you'll likely end up frustrated and overtrained by following their routines. I know all too well—I fell into the same trap early on in my lifting career.

The MAX Muscle Plan is designed for the rest of us. Whether you are new to exercise or a seasoned trainee, the program will help you maximize your muscle potential. No gimmicks. No expensive supplements. All that's required is commitment, dedication, and, of course, a good deal of sweat and effort. This might sound like hyperbole, but I assure you it's not.

How can I be so sure? Because I've successfully used the program with hundreds of private clients over the years. If you follow the protocol as directed, you will get results.

WHAT IS THE MAX MUSCLE PLAN?

The MAX Muscle Plan is a six-month periodized program that systematically manipulates exercise variables to maximize muscle gains. MAX is an acronym for "mitogen-activated xtreme" training. Simply stated, mitogens are chemical substances that encourage cells to remodel—a process that is essential to muscle growth. As the name implies, the ultimate goal of the program is to enhance mitogenic and other growth-oriented training responses in a manner that promotes optimal muscle development.

The thing that sets the MAX Muscle Plan apart from other programs is its scientific approach. I've spent the better part of the past 20 years poring over just about every research paper written on the subject of muscle development. It was my primary focus of interest during my graduate work at the University of Texas and ultimately became the subject of my master's thesis. The culmination of my studies was a comprehensive research review article, "The Mechanisms of Muscle Hypertrophy and Their Application to Resistance Training," which was published in the prestigious *Journal of Strength and Conditioning Research*. I harnessed all of this science, along with years and years of practical experience, to create the MAX Muscle Plan.

Here's how I lay it out in the book.

Chapters 1 and 2 explain the science behind the program. You'll learn how muscles adapt to training and what causes them to grow. Don't worry; I break down the jargon into language that anyone can comprehend. No scientific background is required.

Chapters 3 through 5 detail all the exercises included in the program—more than 100 exercises total. Exercises are described in depth and illustrated in accompanying photos. Expert tips are provided for optimal performance.

Chapters 6 through 9 are the crux of the book: a complete blueprint for achieving your ultimate body. A MAX break-in routine is provided to help those with less than six months of resistance-training experience or those returning to training after a long layoff prepare for the rigors of the three phases of the plan: MAX strength, MAX metabolic, and MAX muscle. Each phase is discussed at length, and every exercise, every set, and every rep is mapped out in explicit detail.

Chapters 10 and 11 address the role of nutrition and cardio in your muscle-building efforts. You'll learn how properly harnessing these factors can help to support muscle development and minimize body fat deposition. Some of the recommendations may come as a surprise, but they're backed up by solid science and years of practical experience.

WHAT RESULTS CAN YOU EXPECT?

The results that you achieve from the MAX Muscle Plan depend on two factors: training status and genetics. If you've been training for less than a year or so, you can expect to see large increases in muscle size. It's not unusual for a novice lifter to gain 15 or more pounds of muscle over the six-month training period. As you gain more training experience, however, results will necessarily slow. This is where the MAX Muscle Plan sets itself apart from other programs. It will help you blast through training plateaus so that you continue to progress in your muscle-building efforts. Using this plan, highly experienced natural bodybuilders have put on an additional 6 to 10 pounds of lean muscle by the end of the training cycle.

Like it or not, genetics also enters into the equation. As the saying goes, you can't escape your gene pool. Don't have great muscle-building genetics? Don't sweat it. Genetics account for only about 25 to 50% of your ultimate potential. That leaves a lot of room for improvement! Although you may have a difficult time becoming the next Mr. Olympia, you unquestionably can develop an impressive physique that is sure to turn heads at the beach. The MAX Muscle Plan will help you squeeze out every ounce of your genetic potential to achieve your best body ever.

I sum things up with my favorite fitness axiom: Exercise is both a science and an art. The MAX Muscle Plan combines science and art into a cohesive system of training that is hands down the most effective muscle-building program on the market. So if you're ready to take your body to the next level, turn the page and read on!

CHAPTER 1

The Science of Muscle Development

The human body is by far the most amazing piece of machinery in the world, capable of incredible feats of strength and intellect. Perhaps its most remarkable attribute, though, is its unique ability to adapt to almost any obstacle it faces. No human-made device comes anywhere close to approximating these adaptive qualities.

That said, the body doesn't like change. Under normal circumstances, it strives to maintain a stable state known as homeostasis. Only when subjected to stress is the body forced to deviate from its homeostatic comfort zone and produce an adaptive response. The muscles are no exception. Just like every other body tissue, they seek to maintain homeostasis. Accordingly, muscle growth takes place only when a stress (such as lifting a weight) is imposed that challenges your muscles beyond their present capacity. This concept, called the principle of overload, is arguably the most important tenet of muscle development. If muscles are not sufficiently overloaded on a regular basis, they have no impetus to develop.

Here's how things play out in the gym. When you lift weights in a manner that challenges your muscles, your body perceives it as a threat to its survival. Your body, in turn, adapts by getting bigger and stronger so that it can effectively deal with the same stimulus when it is encountered in the future. This adaptation—muscle development—continues in this manner as long as you regularly apply physical stresses to overload your muscles.

During the initial stages of training, the primary exercise-related adaptation involves reprogramming your nervous system. Basically, your muscles become more economical at coordinating movement patterns involved in lifting weights. You progress from disorganized, choppy movements to smooth, efficient ones. Over time, your skill level improves until the movements become second nature. This neurological response brings about substantial increases in strength without the benefit of increased muscle size.

Once exercise technique becomes more fluent, usually after a couple months of consistent training, you are able to channel your energies into exerting greater amounts of force during a given lift. At this point your muscles begin to get larger, facilitating further improvements in strength. Muscle growth is achieved by increases in both the size and number of the contractile proteins—actin and myosin—that carry out movement. Contractile proteins are added next to one another in a parallel fashion, like sardines in a tin can. The more contractile proteins you add, the bigger your muscles get.

Muscle growth isn't a one-way street; the process can also work in reverse. Muscle is metabolically active tissue, and its maintenance requires increased caloric expenditure. If you stop working out, your body will perceive unused muscle as energetically wasteful. Your body will thus initiate catabolic (breaking down) processes to get rid of the excess, resulting in a loss of muscle, also known as atrophy. This is known as the principle of reversibility, or "use it or lose it." Although your body seeks homeostasis, it is actually in a constant state of flux that favors muscle atrophy unless you actively engage in challenging muscular activity.

TRIGGERING MUSCLE GROWTH

When it comes to muscle, protein is king. Although water makes up the majority of muscle tissue (approximately 70 percent of muscle weight), it is the protein component (approximately 25 percent of muscle weight) that is responsible for carrying out human movement. The extent of muscle development is predicated on the balance between muscle protein synthesis, or building, and muscle protein breakdown. When synthesis is greater than breakdown, you are in an anabolic (building up) state that's conducive to building muscle.

Contrary to popular belief, you don't build your muscles when you work out. In fact, the opposite actually occurs. Muscle tissue breaks down at an accelerated rate during training, and protein synthesis is largely suppressed. Although this may seem counterintuitive, it is necessary for facilitating bigger, stronger muscles. Compare it to renovating your kitchen. You have to tear out the existing Formica countertops and the pressboard cabinetry before installing the high-end granite and fine hardwood, right? Similarly, outmoded muscle proteins must first be demolished and removed in order to allow newer, better proteins to take their place.

Muscle tissue rebuilds after exercise. During this time, muscle protein synthesis skyrockets and breakdown gradually diminishes. Protein synthesis can remain increased for 48 hours or more postexercise. During this time your muscles supercompensate by growing larger.

The underlying processes responsible for muscle development are highly complex and not well understood. It is generally accepted that the regulation of muscle tissue is carried out, at least in part, through the signaling of various pathways associated with protein synthesis and breakdown. These pathways are diverse and provide a variety of ways for muscle to adapt to overload. The common element of all muscle-building pathways is that they conduct signals through specialized enzymes, setting off a chain of events that ultimately promote protein synthesis and inhibit protein breakdown.

Current research indicates that three primary mechanisms are involved in exercise-related muscle growth: muscle tension, muscle damage, and metabolic stress (Schoenfeld 2010).

1. **Muscle tension.** Tension exerted on muscles during resistance exercise is generally considered the most important factor in muscle development. The tension from lifting weights disturbs the integrity of working muscles, thus bringing about a phenomenon called mechanotransduction. Simply stated, mechanotransduction is the process by which mechanical signals are converted into chemical activity; in this case, the signals turn on anabolic pathways. Up to a certain point, greater muscle tension leads to a greater anabolic stimulus—a classic case of adaptation. However, it seems that an upper limit exists, beyond which high tension levels have a diminishing effect on muscle growth. Once this threshold is reached, other factors become increasingly more important in the growth process. This is why bodybuilders generally display superior muscle growth compared with powerlifters even though bodybuilders routinely train with lighter weights.

2. **Muscle damage.** Anyone who lifts weights has undoubtedly felt achy and sore after an intense exercise session. This phenomenon, called delayed-onset muscle soreness (DOMS), generally manifests approximately 24 hours after an intense workout, and the peak effects are seen about two to three days postexercise. DOMS is caused by localized damage to muscle tissue in the form of microtears in both the contractile proteins and surface membrane (i.e., sarcolemma) of the working muscles. What many people fail to grasp, however, is that a certain amount of soreness may indirectly benefit muscle development. Here's why: The response to muscle damage can be likened to the acute inflammatory response to infection. Once the body perceives damage, immune cells (neutrophils, macrophages, and so on) migrate to the damaged tissue in order to remove cellular debris to help maintain the fiber's ultrastructure. In the process, the body produces signaling molecules called cytokines that activate the release of growth factors involved in muscle development. In this roundabout way, localized inflammation—a source of DOMS—leads to a growth response that,

in effect, strengthens the ability of muscle tissue to withstand future muscle damage. Adaptation!

That said, soreness is by no means a prerequisite for muscle development. Your muscles, connective tissue, and immune system become increasingly efficient in dealing with fiber-related damage associated with intense training (again, an adaptive response). Various physiologic and structural adaptations that take place gradually reduce the sensation of pain. Generally speaking, the more you train at high levels of intensity, the greater your resistance to muscle soreness—even though you invariably inflict damage to fibers. This is why some of the world's top bodybuilders never get sore after a workout, yet display impressive muscularity. Furthermore, too much soreness can actually be detrimental to muscle growth. If you're so sore that it hurts to sit or comb your hair, you've exceeded your body's ability to repair the damaged muscle tissue—and that means you're not growing!

3. **Metabolic stress.** Perhaps the most intriguing factor associated with muscle development is exercise-induced metabolic stress. Research on patients confined to bed rest show that metabolic stress induced by the application of a pressure cuff can help attenuate muscle wasting, even in the absence of exercise. Other studies have found that pressure-cuff exercise performed with very light weights—far less than what is normally considered sufficient for promoting muscular adaptations—can promote significant muscle growth as a result of generating a substantial amount of metabolic stress.

The muscle-building effects of metabolic stress can be attributed to the production of by-products of metabolism called metabolites. These small fragments (including lactate, hydrogen ion, and inorganic phosphate) indirectly mediate cell signaling. Some scientists believe that this is accomplished by increasing water within muscle—a phenomenon known as cell swelling. Studies have shown that cell swelling stimulates protein synthesis and simultaneously decreases protein breakdown. It is not clear exactly why cell swelling causes an anabolic effect, but the prevailing theory suggests a self-preservation mechanism. That is, an increase in water within the cell exerts pressure against the cell wall, similar to overinflating a rubber tire. The cell, in turn, perceives this as a threat to its integrity and responds by sending out anabolic signals that initiate strengthening of its ultrastructure. Adaptation!

Understand that muscle tension, muscle damage, and metabolic stress generally do not exist in isolation. Rather, they combine to produce an additive effect on building lean muscle. Only by achieving an optimal mix of these factors in your training routine can you maximize muscle development.

CALLING ALL SATELLITES

Muscle building is predicated on your body's capacity for protein synthesis; therefore, the relevant machinery must be in place to produce the required muscle proteins. This protein-making machinery is located in the cell nucleus.

Whereas most body tissues have only one nucleus, muscle fibers are multinucleated, meaning that they contain many nuclei. This should make intuitive sense. The majority of cells in the body have a fixed size; however, muscle needs to be able to grow bigger and stronger in response to imposed demands. As you can imagine, this requires a lot of machinery! Compare it to a factory. If you have only a single processing plant, your capacity to produce a given product is limited to the capacity of that one unit. However, add a second plant and you effectively double your production capacity. Add a couple more plants and you increase production fourfold. The more plants, the greater your production capacity.

One little problem, though. As mentioned, the body doesn't like excess. It wants to maintain homeostasis in the manner that is least taxing. Thus, muscle maintains only enough nuclei to meet its present demands for producing protein. Any extra nuclei are deemed superfluous and are discarded. What happens, then, when you begin a workout regimen and suddenly need additional nuclei to make more proteins? Enter the wonder of satellite cells.

Satellite cells are the muscle equivalent of stem cells. These nonspecialized cells reside close to the muscle fiber and remain dormant unless and until strenuous exercise wakes them up. Once aroused, satellite cells go into action. They multiply in number, become more specialized, and fuse to existing muscle fibers to provide the precursor materials needed for repair and subsequent growth of new muscle tissue. Perhaps more importantly, they donate their nuclei to the stimulated muscle fibers so that protein synthesis can increase and support growth.

A study by Petrella and colleagues (2008) from the University of Alabama highlights just how important satellite cells are in maximizing muscle development. The researchers studied the response of 66 adults to 16 weeks of resistance training that focused on the quadriceps muscles. At the end of the study, participants were classified into one of three groups based on the extent of the growth of their quads: extreme responders (average increase of 58 percent in muscle size), moderate responders (average increase of 28 percent in muscle size), and nonresponders (no change in muscle size). Some of the participants achieved tremendous muscle gains whereas others failed to improve at all. One of the most striking reasons for this difference was that both extreme and moderate responders displayed far more satellite cell activity (23 and 19 percent, respectively) than nonresponders. This supports the conclusion that satellite cells are a limiting factor in muscle development and that increasing their activity stimulates greater growth.

THE HORMONE CONNECTION

It doesn't take an exercise scientist to realize that hormones play a substantial role in muscle development. Compare the physique of a juiced-up pro bodybuilder with that of someone who competes naturally. The amount of influence that anabolic hormones can have on muscle size becomes patently apparent. It is not unusual for a person to gain 20 to 30 pounds (10 to 14 kg) in a matter of weeks after going on a steroid cycle. Good luck if you try gaining that naturally.

Interestingly, research shows that intense resistance exercise can cause large hormonal spikes after training. In some cases, increases in hormone levels are of the magnitude of several hundred percent. It therefore seems to make sense that the best exercise routines for muscle growth are those that produce the greatest hormonal response, right? Well, not necessarily.

Understand that pro bodybuilders are essentially walking pharmacies. They take enormous doses of a variety of anabolic hormones that keep hormone levels increased 24/7. The effects of exercise on hormone levels, on the other hand, are transient and generally last for a matter of minutes to hours after a workout. The difference between chronically high hormonal levels and a hormonal spike is the difference between apples and oranges: You just can't compare the two.

Does this then mean that postworkout increases in hormones are irrelevant? Not necessarily. Although research shows that resistance training can increase muscle development in the absence of hormones, spiking hormonal production can potentially magnify muscle-building results. Brief hormonal spikes can act as potent signaling agents, turning on enzymes in the various muscle-building pathways. Once a given enzyme in the pathway is signaled, the cascade of effects proceeds like dominoes falling in a row. Postexercise hormonal increases seem to play at least a permissive role in muscle building, and maximizing their response may augment muscle development.

Numerous hormones and growth factors have been shown to play a role in muscle development. The three most widely studied of these hormones are testosterone, insulin-like growth factor, and growth hormone.

1. **Testosterone.** Widely regarded as the king of all muscle-building hormones, testosterone promotes muscle growth in a variety of ways. First, it directly increases protein synthesis and inhibits protein breakdown. Second, it activates satellite cells, facilitating their effects on muscle tissue. Finally, it can indirectly contribute to protein accretion by stimulating the release of other hormones involved in anabolism. Although these anabolic effects are seen in the absence of exercise, lifting weights magnifies the actions of testosterone. In males, the majority of testosterone is produced in the testes. Women produce only a small fraction of the testosterone of the average male, which is a primary reason why most women find it very difficult to bulk up.

2. **Insulin-like growth factor.** Although testosterone gets most of the publicity when it comes to building muscle, insulin-like growth factor (IGF-1) is perhaps even more important with respect to the direct effects of exercise. Several types of IGF-1 have been identified. Two of these IGF-1 forms—a systemic form that is released primarily by the liver, and a muscle-specific form called mechano growth factor (MGF) that is activated in response to muscle contraction—appear to be particularly relevant to muscle adaptation. Because it is specific to muscle tissue, MGF is considered the more important of the two forms. Current research indicates that the activation of MGF kickstarts muscle growth in a variety of ways, such as increasing the rate of protein synthesis, activating satellite cells, and increasing muscle calcium levels. MGF appears to be especially sensitive to muscle damage, and metabolic stress may enhance levels of MGF.

3. **Growth hormone.** Despite its name, growth hormone (GH) is not nearly as anabolic as either IGF-1 or testosterone. GH is primarily a repartitioning agent. It is involved in increasing the use of fat for fuel as well stimulating the uptake and incorporation of amino acids into various body proteins. GH seems to have a greater effect on reducing body fat than on building muscle. Most of the anabolic effects of GH are likely related to its symbiotic relationship with IGF-1. Specifically, GH preferentially upregulates the production of IGF-1, including the MGF form. Given the importance of IGF-1 in protein synthesis, this may be the most prominent muscle-building role of GH.

The mechanisms of muscle growth are highly complex and involve the intricate signaling of various pathways within the cells. The growth process is supported by satellite cell activity as well as the interaction of various hormones and growth factors. Maximizing these factors requires a training routine that elicits an optimal mix of muscle tension, muscle damage, and metabolic stress. Chapter 2 details exactly how to create such a routine.

CHAPTER 2

MAX Periodization

Ask me what's the most important factor in achieving a terrific physique and, without a second thought, I'll say proper planning. An old adage states, "Those who fail to plan plan to fail." With respect to exercise, never was a saying more apt.

Think of it this way: You wouldn't embark on a road trip without first mapping out your destination, right? If you don't plan your route, you're bound to get lost. Yet, in effect, this is how most people approach their workouts. It's all too common for a trainee to aimlessly wander around the gym thinking, *What should I do now?* Such a haphazard approach is doomed to produce substandard results. To maximize your body's genetic potential, you must individualize a plan that is consistent with your training goals. Each workout must fit into the overall scheme of what you are trying to accomplish and you must properly execute the plan every time you hit the gym.

Central to creating an individualized training plan is the principle of specificity. This principle dictates that the results you get from training are specific to the type of exercise you perform. For example, if you jog for two hours every day, your body will adapt by improving its capacity for aerobic endurance. The quantity of mitochondria in your muscles will increase, as will the activity of various aerobic enzymes. Intense resistance training, on the other hand, leads to improved neural responses and increases in the size of muscle fibers. Bottom line: Whatever your fitness goals, your training program must focus on eliciting adaptations that are specific to these goals.

Planning, however, isn't quite as simple as following a cookie-cutter training routine. One of the biggest mistakes a lifter can make is to perform the same exercises in the same fashion over and over. Ultimately the body gets used to the same old same old, which diminishes the need for future adaptation. What's more, boredom sets in, bringing about a condition called monotonous overtraining that causes a maladaptation of the neuromuscular system. The upshot: Progress slows to a crawl, inevitably leading to a training plateau or, worse, regression.

A BETTER WAY TO PLAN

How can you structure an exercise program that allows you to make ongoing progress and avoid that dreaded training plateau? The solution can be summed up in one word: *periodization*. Originally developed by Russian strength coaches to prepare their athletes for Olympic competition, periodization refers to the systematic manipulation of the variables of an exercise program (reps, sets, rest intervals, and so on) in a manner that optimizes a given fitness component.

The traditional periodized program, commonly known as linear periodization, is divided into three components: macrocycle, mesocycle, and microcycle. The macrocycle customarily represents the entire training year but can vary from several months to up to four years. The macrocycle is subdivided into two or more mesocycles that last from several weeks to several months. Mesocycles are subdivided into microcycles of one to four weeks.

An alternative to the traditional periodization model is undulating periodization. Rather than dividing training cycles over months or years, undulating periodization uses a nonlinear model in which variables are manipulated over short time periods, generally on a week-to-week or even session-to-session basis. If all this periodization talk sounds a bit fuzzy, don't worry. It will all make sense soon.

The basis of periodization can be traced to the General Adaptation Syndrome (GAS)—a theory coined in the 1930s by Austrian scientist Hans Selye. During the course of his research, Selye noticed that the body undergoes a triphasic response to stress. First comes the alarm stage, in which the body responds to a new stress by eliciting an acute fight-or-flight response. With repeated exposure to the stressor, the body enters a resistance stage, in which it supercompensates to deal with the stress. If the stressor persists for an extended time, however, the body becomes unable to adapt and enters the exhaustion stage. Ultimately the body's resources become depleted, resulting in an inability to maintain normal bodily function. This leads to a chronic disease state.

Given that exercise is a potent stressor, the GAS theory is relevant to program design. A training cycle should be continued just long enough to elicit an adaptive response (i.e., the upper edge of the resistance stage). Once this critical point is reached, a new training variable must be introduced in order to sustain progress. At various points throughout the cycle, periods of lower-intensity exercise must be interspersed with periods of higher-intensity exercise to avoid entering the exhaustion stage.

That said, it can be beneficial to occasionally push your body into the exhaustion stage during the course of a periodized routine. Doing so brings about a phenomenon called overreaching. Short-term overreaching can optimize the body's ability to supercompensate, thereby maximizing muscle development. The key is to limit the overreaching to very brief periods, generally no more than a couple weeks. If overreaching persists for too long, it inevitably devolves into overtraining and a corresponding decrease in results.

MAX MUSCLE PLAN: A PERIODIZED APPROACH

The MAX Muscle Plan is a six-month periodized program designed to maximize your muscular potential. This program is a hybrid of the linear and undulating periodization models. Similar to linear periodization, it includes three mesocycles: a MAX strength phase, a MAX metabolic phase, and a MAX muscle phase. But consistent with undulating periodization, it uses a technique called block periodization, in which variables are manipulated on a weekly basis. Several training variables are manipulated: intensity, volume, rest intervals, effort, tempo, frequency, and exercise selection.

Intensity

Training intensity is arguably the most important exercise variable for muscle development, at least up to a point. For our purposes, the term intensity refers to the amount of weight lifted rather than the amount of effort put into the lift. Intensity is generally measured as a percentage of repetition maximum (RM). Simply stated, RM is the maximal amount of weight you can lift a given number of times with good form. A 1RM equals the amount of weight you can lift once but not a second time; a 10RM is the weight you can lift 10 times but not 11. The weight used for a given exercise must be heavy enough to recruit and fatigue the full spectrum of muscle fibers; if not, muscle development will be suboptimal.

Training intensity dictates the number of repetitions that you can perform for a particular exercise. This is called the repetition range. Repetitions can be classified into three approximate ranges: low (1 to 5), moderate (6 to 12), and high (15 or more). Each of these repetition ranges involves the use of different energy systems and taxes the neuromuscular system in different ways.

A low repetition range (approximately 90 to 100 percent 1RM) is best for increasing muscle strength. This should make intuitive sense given that strength is defined as the ability to exert maximal force. Because training in a low rep range maximizes gains in strength, people often assume that lifting near-maximal weight is the best way to increase muscle size. It's not. Sure, muscles are under a lot of tension during a low-rep set. But the limited time under tension shortchanges stimulation to certain fibers, reducing the potential for microtrauma, or small degrees of muscle damage. Moreover, because low-rep sets last a very short time—typically less than 15 seconds— little if any metabolic stress is generated. Bottom line: Although performing low-rep sets will certainly lead to muscle growth, it's not an ideal way to maximize muscular gains.

At the other end of the intensity spectrum, a high rep range of less than about 60 percent 1RM is associated with adaptations specific to local muscular endurance (i.e., the ability to lift submaximal weights multiple times) with diminished effects on muscle growth. From a muscle-development standpoint, this represents the opposite of low-rep training. Although working in a high rep range does generate a significant amount of metabolic stress, the tension on muscles is inadequate for recruiting and fatiguing fast-twitch muscle fibers—the ones with the greatest growth potential (see Muscle Fiber Types in the next section).

By now you've probably guessed that training in a moderate rep range of approximately 65 to 85 percent 1RM is optimal for building muscle. This is consistent with the theory that a maximum threshold for tension-induced hypertrophy exists, above which metabolic factors become more important than additional increases in load. Moderate reps provide an ideal mix of these factors. For one, the weights are heavy enough to generate significant muscle tension. What's more, the tension is maintained for a sufficient time to enhance the potential for microtrauma and fatigability across the full spectrum of available fibers in working muscles.

Moderate-rep schemes also generate a significant buildup of metabolites that enhance the body's anabolic environment, setting the stage for muscle growth. As discussed in chapter 1, a by-product of metabolite production is cell swelling, commonly referred to as a muscle pump. People often dismiss the pump as a temporary cosmetic phenomenon, but this dismissal is short sighted. Recall that the body perceives cell swelling as a threat to the integrity of the affected muscle fibers. The body responds by increasing protein synthesis and decreasing protein breakdown—the basis of muscle development.

The MAX Muscle Plan makes use of a technique called step loading, in which progressive increases in intensity are followed by a brief period of unloading. This structure creates a wavelike loading pattern that allows the use of a broad spectrum of reps within a target rep range while reducing the potential for overtraining. You'll see how this plays out in the training chapters.

Volume

Training volume runs a close second to intensity in terms of importance to muscle growth, and it may play an even greater role for experienced lifters. Simply stated, workout volume is the amount of exercise you perform over a given time (usually expressed on weekly basis). Volume is determined by adding up the total number of repetitions performed in a training session. Some fitness pros also factor in the amount of weight lifted, but this approach can be misleading in a routine designed for muscle development. For our purposes, we'll keep it simple and define volume as total repetitions.

Muscle Fiber Types

The two basic types of muscle fibers are slow twitch (Type I) and fast twitch (Type II). Slow-twitch fibers are endurance-oriented fibers that can withstand repeated contractions but have a limited ability to generate force. Fast-twitch fibers, on the other hand, have a substantial capacity for generating force but tend to fatigue easily.

As you probably expect from these descriptions, fast-twitch fibers have a significantly greater capacity for growth than slow-twitch fibers—about 50 percent greater by most accounts. Some lifters mistakenly take this to mean that slow-twitch fibers do not get bigger. Not true. Although slow-twitch fibers are not as responsive to growth as fast-twitch fibers, they nevertheless do hypertrophy when subjected to an overload stimulus. Given that the majority of whole muscles comprise a significant number of slow-twitch fibers, regardless of individual variance, this can potentially help maximize whole-muscle girth.

Interestingly, studies show that bodybuilders display greater hypertrophy of slow-twitch fibers than do powerlifters. This apparently is due to differences in training methodology—bodybuilders train with higher reps than powerlifters—and seems to explain, at least in part, why bodybuilders are more muscular than powerlifters.

Given that reps are carried out in sets, training volume is predicated on the number of sets you perform in a workout. Traditional lifting protocols, which date to the classic Delorme-Watkins method developed in the late 1940s, advocated performing three sets of each exercise in a workout. For decades thereafter this was considered standard advice. Beginning in the early 1970s, however, some in the fitness field began to challenge the wisdom of multiple-set training. Arthur Jones, founder of Nautilus, is credited as the first to put forth the notion that only a single set is required for stimulating growth. Jones argued that as long as a set is performed to muscle failure, any additional sets are superfluous and are actually counterproductive to muscle development. This theory, which came to be known as high-intensity training (HIT), was soon embraced by Mike Mentzer, Ellington Darden, and other notables in the industry. Today, HIT continues to enjoy a large following within a subset of the lifting population.

Does HIT work? Absolutely. Provided that you train sufficiently hard, an HIT routine increases strength and builds muscle. For those pressed for time, it can be an efficient alternative to multi-set training.

That said, higher-volume protocols have consistently proven superior to single-set protocols when it comes to maximizing muscle strength and hypertrophy. And we're not talking slight differences here. A meta-analysis reported

46 percent greater increases in strength and 40 percent greater increases in muscle growth when multiple-set protocols were compared with single-set protocols (Krieger 2010). It's not entirely clear whether this superiority is the product of greater total muscle tension, muscle damage, metabolic stress, or some combination of these factors. One thing, however, is patently clear: If you want to make the most of your muscular potential, multiple-set routines are a must.

How many sets are optimal? Anywhere from two to four sets per exercise is generally a good guideline, although this can vary somewhat depending on program design. Keep in mind, though, that long workouts tend to be associated with reduced intensity of effort, decreased motivation, and alterations in immune response. Thus, it's generally best to limit intensive workouts to no longer than an hour in length to ensure maximal training capacity throughout each lifting session. What's more, consistently training with high volumes can hasten the onset of overtraining. This speaks to the need to vary workout volume across the training cycle so that your body is not taxed beyond its recuperative capacity.

Rest Interval

The amount of time you take from the end of one set to the beginning of the next is called the rest interval. Most lifters give little thought to this variable. They'll meander around between sets with no regard for time. Big mistake. The duration of rest intervals significantly affects muscle tension and metabolite buildup—key elements in muscle development. Make no mistake: Resting too long or too short will negatively affect your results.

Rest intervals can be classified into three broad categories: short (approximately 30 seconds or less), moderate (about 1 to 2 minutes), and long (approximately 3 minutes or more). Long rest intervals allow for complete muscular recovery after performance of a set. You need approximately three minutes between sets to fully regain your strength on a given exercise. Full recovery allows you to train with your heaviest weight within a given repetition range, ensuring that you generate maximal muscle tension during the ensuing set. This level of recovery is good for increasing both strength and size. On the other hand, any metabolite buildup that may arise dissipates over the course of the rest period, which is good for strength but not for size. Bottom line: Longer rest intervals are beneficial when your goal is to enhance basic strength, but they are not ideal for maximizing muscle growth.

Short rest intervals basically have the opposite effect. Metabolite accumulation skyrockets with limited rest periods. Not only does this enhance the body's anabolic environment, it makes your muscles more impervious to lactic acid—factors beneficial for both muscular endurance and size. The downside is that short rest intervals do not allow sufficient time to regain your strength. In fact, strength decrements of up to 50 percent are seen in subsequent sets when rest intervals are limited to 30 seconds. The result is that muscle tension is compromised, making it difficult to build substantial amounts of muscle.

Moderate rest intervals offer an effective compromise for enhancing muscle development. For one thing, a majority of your strength—enough to generate substantial muscular tension—is recaptured following a moderate rest period. Better yet, consistently training with moderate rest intervals leads to adaptations that ultimately allow you to sustain performance with even higher percentages of your RM—up to 90 percent of maximal strength capacity for a given RM. Moderate rest intervals also promote significant metabolic stress, particularly when combined with moderate repetitions. Large spikes in metabolite production are seen following such exercise protocols, enhancing anabolic signaling. From a muscle-building standpoint, moderate rest intervals represent the best of both worlds.

Effort

The effort you expend during a set will significantly affect your results. Muscle gains come only by stressing your muscles beyond their present capacity. This is a basic application of the overload principle, which is discussed in chapter 1. If you don't challenge your muscles, they have no impetus to grow. Period.

One of the most controversial topics among fitness professionals is whether it is beneficial to train to momentary muscle failure—the point during a set when muscles can no longer produce enough force to complete the lift. In one camp are those who claim you should reach failure on every set of every exercise. In another camp are those who say failure is unnecessary and even counterproductive to results. Who's right? If the goal is muscle development, the answer seems to lie somewhere between the two extreme positions.

On one hand, training to failure can increase recruitment of muscle fibers. When a lifter becomes fatigued, a progressively greater number of fibers are recruited to continue muscular activity, providing an additional stimulus for muscle growth. Perhaps more importantly, recruited fibers are subjected to high degrees of tension for a greater period, ensuring their optimal stimulation and microtrauma.

When moderate to high reps are used, training to failure also may enhance exercise-induced metabolic stress. Studies show that increases in anabolic hormone are greater when sets are performed to failure than when they are not performed to failure (Willardson, Norton, and Wilson, 2010). You don't have to be an exercise scientist to know that you get a greater pump—which is indicative of a high degree of cell swelling—when you go all out in a set. These acute effects are associated with greater protein synthesis and thus increased muscle growth.

The downside of training to muscle failure is that the potential for overtraining and psychological burnout increases. Reductions in resting testosterone and insulin-like growth factor concentrations—widely used markers of overtraining—have been reported when lifters repeatedly trained to failure over a 16-week period. Thus, although some failure training is necessary to maximize muscle development, too much is destined to have a negative effect.

How much is too much? Tough to say. Some lifters can tolerate failure training more readily than others. The key is to periodize this variable over the course of a training cycle. If any signs of overtraining manifest, reduce the frequency of sets performed to failure accordingly.

How do you quantify effort if you don't train to failure? A simple method is to use a rating of perceived exertion (RPE). Although several RPE scales exist, for the resistance training outlined in this book we use a scale of 1 to 10. See table 2.1 for an RPE scale you can use to gauge effort during resistance training.

Table 2.1 10-Point Resistance Training RPE Scale

Rating	Effort level
1	Complete rest
2	Extremely easy
3	Very easy
4	Easy
5	Moderate
6	Somewhat hard
7	Hard
8	Very hard
9	Extremely hard
10	Muscular failure

Tempo

Tempo refers to the speed with which you perform a repetition. It is specific to the three types of contractions: concentric, eccentric, and isometric. The concentric, or positive, portion of a lift occurs when you lift a weight against the force of gravity; the eccentric, or negative, portion of a lift occurs when you lower a weight in the direction of gravity; and the isometric, or static, portion of a lift occurs when the weight is not moving up or down. For example, the concentric portion of a biceps curl takes place when you bring the bar up toward your shoulders. Alternatively, lowering the bar constitutes the eccentric phase of the lift. The isometric phase occurs at the top position and bottom portion of the lift because the weight is stationary at these points.

Tempo can be expressed as a four-digit number, separated by hyphens, in which the first number represents the concentric phase, the second number the isometric phase at the top of the lift, the third number the eccentric phase, and the fourth number the isometric phase at the bottom of the lift. In the example of the biceps curl, a tempo of 1-0-3-0 means that the concentric phase lasts 1 second, the isometric phase at the top of the lift is imperceptible, the eccentric phase lasts 3 seconds, and the isometric phase at the bottom of the lift is imperceptible.

How fast (or slow, depending on your perspective) should you lift? With respect to concentric repetitions, the best advice is to lift explosively. Provided that you maintain control throughout the lift, try to move the weight as quickly as possible. This generally results in speeds of one to two seconds to complete the concentric action. (You will necessarily perform the last few reps of a set more slowly than the first few reps as a result of increased muscle fatigue, but the intent is always to lift in explosive fashion.)

Superslow Training

The technique of superslow training has gained some popularity in recent years. In this form of resistance exercise training, each repetition takes about 15 seconds to complete. It is based on the concept that performing repetitions at an extremely slow tempo reduces momentum and therefore increases force to the target muscle. In addition, by reducing momentum, the potential for injury is supposedly decreased. Although this may sound logical, closer examination suggests otherwise.

First, the effects of momentum on training are wildly overstated. Provided that weights are lifted in a controlled fashion, the target muscles perform the majority of the work. Momentum is not a factor. What's more, simply slowing the speed of repetitions has no effect on reducing injuries. In fact, the injury rate for those who train with proper form and technique in a traditional protocol is almost nonexistent. Thus, the science behind the superslow claims simply doesn't add up.

In addition to being an extremely tedious form of training, superslow training is suboptimal for achieving maximal muscle development. Here's why. First, the weights used during superslow training must be extremely light to compensate for the slow speed of the lift. Although this allows the concentric portion of the rep to be executed in the desired fashion, it takes away most of the muscular stress on the eccentric portion. (Muscles can handle significantly more weight on eccentric actions than on concentric actions.) Because the eccentric component is perhaps the most important aspect in promoting muscle development, superslow training simply can't compare with performing reps at a traditional cadence.

A somewhat slower tempo is beneficial on the eccentric portion of a repetition. As a general rule, this phase should take about two to three seconds. Understand that eccentric exercise is perhaps even more important to the growth response than concentric contractions. Here's why. Eccentric actions involve lengthening a muscle under tension, which results in a preferential recruitment of fast-twitch fibers. Because fewer fibers are called on to produce force during eccentric movement, those that are active are forced to bear a greater amount of tension. As a result, microtrauma is increased, leading to greater remodeling of muscle tissue. The take-away message is to resist gravity when lowering the weight. If you don't, you're missing out on more than half of the muscle-building benefits of the exercise!

The isometric portion of the lift is less of a concern from a muscle-development standpoint. Some fitness pros recommend holding the top phase of the lift for a second or so to generate a peak muscular contraction. Research to support such a practice, however, is lacking. Your best bet is to maintain constant tension on the target muscle by not locking out the joint at the top of the lift. Provided that you perform each rep in a smooth, controlled fashion, eliciting a peak isometric contraction is superfluous.

Frequency

Frequency of training refers to the number of exercise sessions you perform in a given period of time (usually reported on a weekly basis). As a general rule, at least three resistance training sessions per week are necessary to maximize muscle development, but a greater frequency can potentially augment results, at least up to a given point. Train too frequently for too long and overtraining ultimately sets in. You can optimize results by periodizing training frequency so that you push your body to the brink without going over the edge.

Another important consideration with respect to training frequency is how much time to allow between sessions that train the same muscle group. Of particular relevance here is the time course of protein synthesis. After an exercise session, protein synthesis is markedly increased. This increase lasts for about 36 to 48 hours postexercise.

Training a muscle group before protein synthesis has completed its course can impair muscular gains. Compare the process to getting a tan. If you are very light skinned and bake in the hot sun for an hour, you are going to burn. In this case, you surely wouldn't go back to the beach the next day because that would only make the burn worse. The burn will subside only if you take a break from the sun. Better yet, your skin adapts during this break by producing more melanin so that the next time it's exposed to the sun you tan instead of burn.

As with a sunburn, going back to the gym before the repair process has fully run its course interferes with the adaptation process. In effect, by not allowing sufficient recovery time you keep breaking down the muscle at a greater rate than the body can rebuild it. The muscle can't keep up with the needed amount of protein synthesis, which hastens the onset of localized overtraining.

Shortchanging the recuperative process also has a negative effect on your strength levels. Studies show that force production is decreased for up to 72 hours after high-intensity resistance workouts (Logan and Abernethy 1996). This reduces the amount of weight you can lift, decreasing muscular tension and thus impairing muscle development.

Taking all factors into account, allow a minimum of 48 hours between exercise sessions that work the same muscle group. Also take into account the recovery of secondary muscles that have played a strong role. Exercises such as pull-downs and rows require substantial muscle contribution from the elbow flexors (biceps brachii), and pressing movements involve a significant contribution from the elbow extensors (triceps brachii). Structure your routines to give adequate recovery time to all muscles receiving significant work in a session. Otherwise, you run the risk of localized overtraining of the involved muscles.

Also note that exercise frequency has a direct effect on total training volume. Assuming that volume within each session remains constant, more frequent workouts will necessarily increase weekly training volume. It therefore follows that, all other things being equal, increased training frequency increases the potential for overtraining. Thus, it's unwise to continue to train on successive days over long periods of time, even if individual muscles are afforded sufficient rest between workout sessions.

To an extent, training frequency is limited by how you structure your routine. Specifically, you can train either in a total-body fashion in which you work all the major muscles in a single session or by various types of split routines in which you perform multiple exercises for a given number of muscle groups in a session. A benefit of total-body training is that each muscle is trained with a greater frequency than in split routines. This is particularly advantageous when the goal is to enhance strength and metabolic adaptations.

Total-body routines generally don't work quite as well when the goal is to maximize muscle development. Compared with full-body routines, a split routine allows you to maintain total weekly training volume while performing fewer sets per training session and affording greater recovery between sessions. This may enable you to use heavier daily training loads and thus generate greater muscular tension. Moreover, split routines can increase metabolic stress by prolonging the training stimulus within a given muscle group, thereby increasing acute anabolic hormone secretions, cell swelling, and muscle ischemia.

Understanding Overtraining

Overtraining is a common exercise-related affliction that affects up to 10 percent of all people who exercise on a regular basis. Because people lack understanding of the subject, it often ends up going undiagnosed.

Simply stated, overtraining results from performing too much strenuous physical activity. However, the exact threshold for overtraining varies from person to person. Some people can tolerate high training volumes and intensities whereas others begin to develop symptoms of overtraining from doing much less. What's more, factors such as nutrition status, sleeping patterns, hormone and enzyme concentrations, muscle fiber composition, and previous training experience all affect recuperative capacity and, therefore, the point at which overtraining rears its ugly head.

Overtraining can be classified into two categories: localized and systemic. Although both have the same origin (too much exercise), their repercussions are quite different. Of the two subtypes, localized overtraining is by far the most common. As the name implies, it is localized to a specific muscle or muscle group and does not affect other body systems. It typically strikes those who are involved in serious strength training programs, especially powerlifters and physique athletes.

Localized overtraining is likely to occur when the same muscle group is trained too frequently in a given time span. This can happen even in a split routine, in which different muscle groups are trained on different days. During the performance of most exercises, a synergistic, or collaborative, interaction occurs between muscle groups. For example, the biceps are integrally involved in the performance of back maneuvers, the shoulders and triceps are involved in many exercises for the chest, and the glutes and hamstrings are involved in many compound leg movements. Other muscles function as stabilizers. The abdominals and erector spinae (the muscles of the lower back), in particular, help provide stability in a variety of upper- and lower-body exercises, contracting statically throughout each move. The fact is that when a muscle is repeatedly subjected to intense physical stress—even on a secondary level—without being afforded adequate rest, the rate at which microtrauma occurs outpaces the reparation process. The end result is impaired localized muscle development.

Systemic overtraining, on the other hand, is more complex and potentially more serious than localized overtraining. As the name implies, it acts on the body as a whole. Commonly referred to as overtraining syndrome (OTS), it affects thousands of people each year.

In almost all cases, OTS causes the body to enter a catabolic state. Catabolism is mediated by an increased production of cortisol—a stress hormone secreted by the adrenal cortex—which exerts its influence at the cellular level, impeding muscular repair and function. Making matters worse, a corresponding decrease often occurs in testosterone production, depleting the body of its most potent anabolic stimulus. Together, these factors combine to inhibit protein synthesis and accelerate proteolysis (protein breakdown). Not only does this result in a cessation of muscle development, it makes the body less efficient at utilizing fat for fuel—a double whammy that wreaks havoc on body composition.

In addition, because of a depletion of glutamine stores, OTS suppresses the body's immune system. Glutamine is the major source of energy for immune cells, and a steady supply of glutamine is necessary for their proper function. However, glutamine levels are rapidly exhausted when exercise volume is high. Without an adequate amount of fuel, the immune system loses its ability to produce antibodies such as lymphocytes, leukocytes, and cytokines. Ultimately, the body's capacity to fight viral and bacterial infections becomes impaired, leading to an increased incidence of infirmity.

Here are some of the symptoms related to overtraining. If you experience two or more of these symptoms, you very well might be overtrained. If symptoms persist, get plenty of sleep and don't resume training until you feel mentally and physically ready.

- Increased resting heart rate
- Increased resting blood pressure
- Decreased exercise performance
- Decreased appetite
- Decreased desire to work out
- Increased incidence of injuries
- Increased incidence of infections and flulike symptoms
- Increased irritability and depression

Exercise Selection

Exercise selection refers to the assortment of exercises you perform in a training routine. Varying exercises is essential to muscle development for several reasons. First, muscles often have different attachment sites (where muscles attach to bone). Depending on the exercise performed, the point of attachment may increase leverage in one aspect of the muscle while decreasing leverage in another aspect. For example, the trapezius (a large muscle in the back) is subdivided so that the upper aspect elevates the scapula, the middle aspect abducts the scapula, and the lower portion depresses the scapula. Hence, shrugs primarily work the upper traps, rows the middle traps, and lat pull-downs the lower traps. Other muscles such as the pectoralis major (the primary chest muscle), deltoids, and triceps are segmented into distinct heads, and each head is responsible for carrying out different joint actions. Thus, an assortment of exercises ensures complete stimulation of all fibers.

Additionally, muscle fibers don't necessarily span the entire length of the muscle as is commonly believed. The rectus abdominis, for example, is subdivided by several fibrous bands called tendinous inscriptions (the connective tissue that gives the abs their six-pack appearance), and the upper and lower segments are supplied by different nerve branches. Other muscles such as the sartorius, gracilis, and various aspects of the hamstrings are similarly subdivided by one or more fibrous bands and innervated by separate nerves. These architectural differences allow you to selectively target portions of a muscle by performing specific movements.

Bottom line: No single exercise can effectively maximize development of a muscle. You can achieve full development only by varying exercise selection so that muscles are worked from different angles in all planes of movement. Moreover, you must frequently rotate exercises to ensure stimulation of the full spectrum of muscle fibers. Even changing hand spacing or foot stance in a movement can bring about different muscular adaptations, thus improving symmetry and development.

Exercises can be classified into two broad categories: multijoint and single joint. Multijoint exercises require two or more joints to carry out the movement. An example is the bench press, in which the shoulder and elbow joints are both involved to lift the weight. Single-joint exercises require movement of only one joint to complete a repetition. An example is the biceps curl, in which the elbow joint is solely responsible for lifting the weight. Both single- and multijoint exercises have a place in a muscle-building routine.

How often should you change exercises? This really depends on the phase of the periodization cycle. Strength improvements tend to be maximized with a limited number of exercises because maximal strength is highly dependent on neuromuscular factors involving the connection between the brain, nervous system, and muscles. The goal is to hardwire the movements into your neural circuitry. The more frequently you perform a given exercise, the more your body develops an affinity for the movement.

During a hypertrophy cycle, on the other hand, frequent rotation of exercises is highly desirable. The goal is to vary parameters such as angle of pull, exercise modality, and so on to elicit different activation patterns within whole muscles and muscle compartments and to provide a unique stimulus to muscle fibers that heightens microtrauma. It can be beneficial to switch up your exercises on a weekly basis. At the very least, aim to switch around your exercises every few weeks or so.

Unstable Surfaces

Wobble boards, Swiss balls, DynaDiscs, BOSU, and other unstable-surface devices are among the most popular pieces of gym equipment. Their use has skyrocketed over the years. Some proponents have gone as far as to claim that every exercise should be performed on an unstable surface. Although these implements can help you attain certain fitness goals, their use is generally not warranted in a muscle-building routine.

From a muscle-building standpoint, the perceived benefit of unstable surface training is actually its biggest weakness. Lifting weights on an unstable surface requires extensive activation of the core musculature. More core activation sounds like a good thing, right? When you consider the tradeoff, it isn't. The increased involvement of the muscles of the abs and lower back comes at the expense of the prime movers (agonists)—you simply can't lift as much weight when training on an unstable surface. Studies show that force output is as much as 70 percent lower when performing exercises on an unstable surface than when performing exercises on a stable surface (Behm, Anderson, and Curnew 2002). Such large reductions in force output diminish dynamic tension to the target muscles, impairing hypertrophic adaptations.

An exception is that the use of unstable surfaces in exercises that directly work the core musculature can be beneficial in a hypertrophy-oriented routine. This makes perfect sense because unstable surfaces increase core activation. The abs in particular can benefit from unstable-surface training. Studies show that crunches performed on a Swiss ball elicit significantly greater muscle activity in the upper and lower rectus abdominis and the external obliques than crunches performed under stable conditions (Sternlicht et al. 2007). Thus, adding in some unstable-surface exercises for direct ab work can only enhance muscle development.

GETTING STARTED

You now have all the background necessary to begin the MAX Muscle Plan. The program is laid out to take all the guesswork out of training. I provide sample routines for every week of each phase of the program. Exercises, sets, reps, and rest intervals are listed in chart form for easy reference. All you have to do is put in the dedication and effort.

Note that the sample routines are a general blueprints for structuring your routine. Consistent with the principle of individuality, adjust exercise variables to better suit your muscle fiber type, psychological stresses, age, training experience, health status, and recovery rate. The best advice I can give is to remain in tune with your body and be willing to experiment according to your individual response.

Also note that the exercises provided in the routines are merely suggestions. If a certain movement doesn't feel right to you or if you don't have access to a particular piece of equipment, then simply substitute a different exercise. Just make sure the replacement is comparable to the one listed, targeting similar muscles in the same plane of movement. Say, for example, that a particular routine calls for a barbell bench press but you don't have access to an Olympic bar or the necessary number of plates. No problem. Perform a dumbbell bench press instead. Although the two exercises are not identical, they work essentially the same muscles in similar ways.

Stoked to begin the routine? Great! Lace up your sneakers, put on your sweats, and let's get started.

CHAPTER 3

Exercises for the Back, Chest, and Abdomen

This chapter describes and illustrates exercises for the chest, back, and abdominal muscles. The back and chest are made up of the most powerful muscles in the upper body. Development of this musculature will ultimately delineate the shape of your physique and enhance your ability to carry out a majority of pulling and pushing movements performed in the course of everyday life. The attributes of a well-developed midsection are readily apparent. Plain and simple, your abdominals are the centerpiece of your body; no muscle group gets more attention. And although body fat levels need to be low in order to see abdominal definition, the often elusive "six-pack" can only be attained by building up the musculature in this region.

Read over the descriptions carefully and scrutinize the photos to ensure proper form. I provide training tips for each of these movements to optimize training performance. Remember that exercises are merely tools for achieving a means to an end—in this case, muscle development. If an exercise does not feel right to you, simply substitute a comparable move.

Dumbbell Pullover

Target

This move targets the lats and middle part of the chest.

Start

Lie on a flat bench so that your upper back rests on the bench and plant your feet firmly on the floor. Grasp a dumbbell with both hands and raise it directly over your face.

Movement

Keeping your elbows slightly bent, slowly lower the dumbbell behind your head as far as comfortably possible. When you feel a complete stretch in your lats, reverse the direction and return to the start position.

Brad's Training Tips

■ Stretch only to the point of comfort—overstretching can lead to shoulder injury.

■ Bend your elbows slightly throughout the move. Do not straighten your elbows as you lift—this increases triceps activation at the expense of your target muscles.

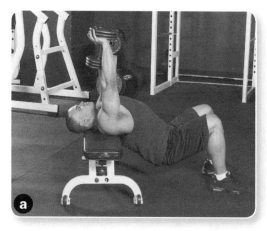
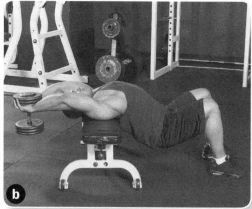

Dumbbell One-Arm Row

Target

This move targets the back muscles and is especially effective for developing the inner-back musculature.

Start

Place your left hand and left knee on a flat bench and plant your right foot firmly on the floor. Grasp a dumbbell in your right hand with your palm facing your body and let the dumbbell hang by your side.

Movement

Keeping your elbow close to your body, pull the dumbbell up and back until it touches your hip. Contract the muscles in your upper back. Reverse the direction and slowly return to the start position. After you complete the desired number of reps on your right side, reposition yourself on the bench and perform the exercise with your left arm.

Brad's Training Tips

- Keep your back slightly arched and your torso parallel to the floor throughout the move.
- Keep your chin up at all times—this helps prevent rounding of the spine.

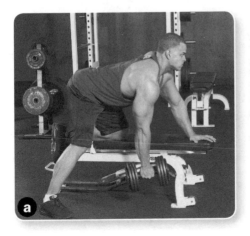

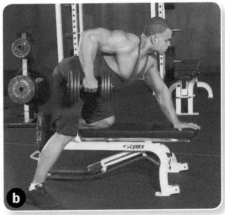

T-Bar Row

Target

This move targets the back muscles.

Start

Stand in a T-bar row apparatus with your feet approximately shoulder-width apart. Bend your knees and place the bar between your legs. Grasp the upper portion of the bar with both hands, one hand above the other, and allow the bar to hang down in front of your body. Bend forward slightly at your hips and hold your core tight.

Movement

Keeping your elbows close to your sides, pull the bar up into your midsection as high as possible. Contract the muscles in your upper back. Reverse the direction and slowly return to the start position.

Brad's Training Tips

- It's extremely important to maintain a slight hyperextension of the lower back. Bending the spine forward can result in lumbar injury.
- Keep your head up at all times—this helps prevent rounding of the spine.
- If you wish to perform this exercise at home, wrap a towel around one end of a barbell and wedge the bar in the corner of the room. The towel will help prevent damage to the wall.

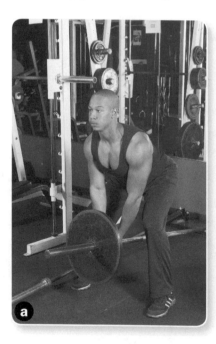 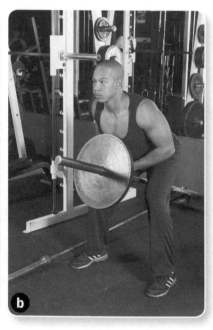

Barbell Reverse-Grip Bent Row

Target

This move targets the back muscles.

Start

Grasp a barbell with your hands shoulder-width apart and your palms facing away from your body. Stand with your body angled forward. Bend your knees and slightly arch your lower back. Allow your arms to hang straight down from your shoulders.

Movement

Keeping your elbows close to your sides, pull the bar up into your midsection as high as possible. Contract the muscles in your upper back. Reverse the direction and slowly return to the start position.

Brad's Training Tips

■ It's extremely important to maintain a slight hyperextension of the lower back. Bending the spine forward can result in lumbar injury.

■ Keep your head up at all times—this helps prevent rounding of the spine.

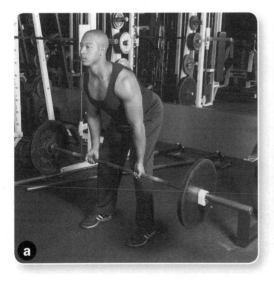

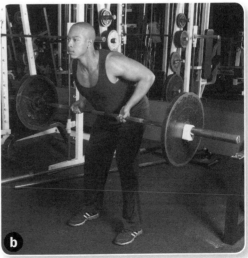

Barbell Overhand Bent Row

Target

This move targets the back muscles.

Start

Grasp a barbell with a shoulder-width grip with your palms facing your body. Slightly angle your body forward, bend your knees, and slightly arch your lower back. Allow your arms to hang straight down from your shoulders.

Movement

Keeping your elbows close to your sides, pull the bar up into your midsection as high as possible. Contract the muscles in your upper back. Reverse the direction and slowly return to the start position.

Brad's Training Tips

- It's extremely important to maintain a slight hyperextension of the lower back. Bending the spine forward can result in lumbar injury.
- Keep your head up at all times—this helps prevent rounding of the spine.

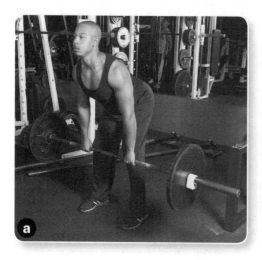

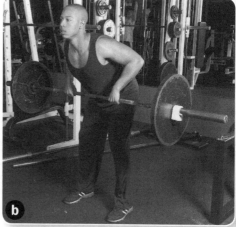

Machine Close-Grip Seated Row

Target

This move targets the back muscles, particularly the inner musculature of the rhomboids and the middle traps.

Start

Sit with your body facing the pad of a seated row machine. Press your chest against the pad and grasp the machine handles with your palms facing each other. Adjust the seat height so that, when you grasp the handles, your arms are fully extended and you feel a stretch in your lats.

Movement

Keeping your elbows close to your sides and your lower back slightly arched, pull the handles back as far as possible without discomfort. Squeeze your shoulder blades together. Reverse the direction and slowly return to the start position.

Brad's Training Tip

- Don't swing your body forward at the beginning of the move—this common mistake overstresses the lower-back muscles and injects unnecessary momentum into the move.

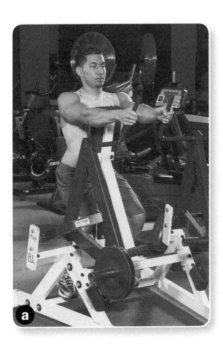
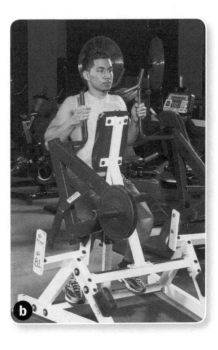

Machine Wide-Grip Seated Row

Target

This move targets the back muscles and posterior deltoid.

Start

Sit with your body facing the pad of a seated row machine. Press your chest against the pad and grasp the machine handles with a wide grip. Adjust the seat height so that, when you grasp the handles, your arms are fully extended and you feel a stretch in your lats.

Movement

Keeping your elbows flared and your lower back slightly arched, pull the handles back as far as possible without discomfort. Squeeze your shoulder blades together. Reverse the direction and slowly return to the start position.

Brad's Training Tip

- Don't swing your body forward at the beginning of the move—this common mistake overstresses the lower-back muscles and injects unnecessary momentum into the move.

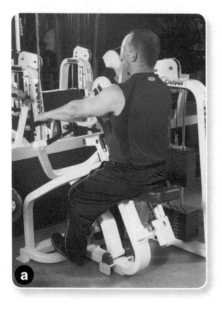 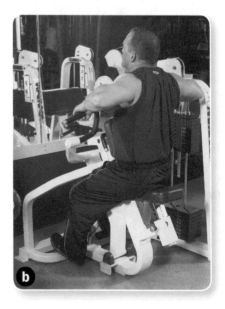

Cable Seated Row

Target

This move targets the back muscles, particularly the inner musculature of the rhomboids and the middle traps.

Start

With your palms facing each other, grasp the handles of a V-bar attached to a low-pulley apparatus. Sit on the seat (or the floor, depending on the unit) and place your feet against the foot plate or a stable part of the unit. Fully straighten your arms so that you feel a complete stretch in your lats. Make sure your posture is erect and slightly arch your lower back.

Movement

Maintaining a slight bend in your knees, pull the handles in toward your lower abdomen, keeping your elbows close to your sides and your lower back tight. Squeeze your shoulder blades together when the handles touch your body. Reverse the direction and slowly return to the start position.

Brad's Training Tips

- Don't lean forward on the return—this interjects momentum into the move on the concentric action, reducing tension to the target muscles.
- Never round your spine—this places the discs in a precarious position and can lead to serious injury.
- You can perform this move with a variety of handle attachments, such as the V-bar and the curved bar.

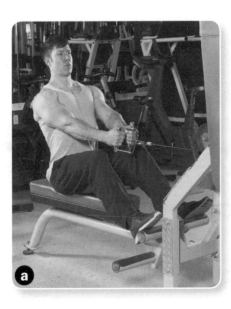 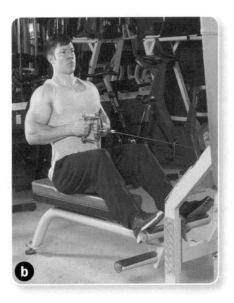

Cable Wide-Grip Seated Row

Target

This move targets the back muscles and posterior deltoid.

Start

With your palms facing each other, grasp the handles of a wide bar attached to a low-pulley apparatus. Sit on the seat (or the floor, depending on the unit) and place your feet against the foot plate or a stable part of the unit. Fully straighten your arms so that you feel a complete stretch in your lats. Make sure your posture is erect and slightly arch your lower back.

Movement

Maintaining a slight bend in your knees, pull the bar in toward your body, keeping your lower back tight. Squeeze your shoulder blades together when the bar touches your body. Reverse the direction and slowly return to the start position.

Brad's Training Tips

- Don't lean forward on the return—this interjects momentum into the move on the concentric action, reducing tension to the target muscles.
- Never round your spine—this places the discs in a precarious position and can lead to serious injury.

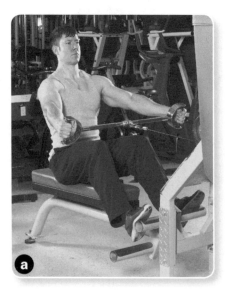
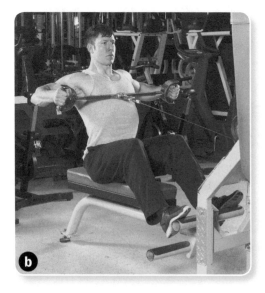

Cable One-Arm Standing Low Row

Target

This move targets the back muscles.

Start

With your palm facing in, grasp the loop handle of a low pulley with your right hand. Step back from the machine and straighten your right arm so that you feel a stretch in your right lat. Keep your right leg back and bend your left leg so that your weight is forward. Brace your left hand against a sturdy part of the unit for support.

Movement

Keeping your elbow close to your body, pull the loop handle toward your right side. Contract your right lat. Reverse the direction and slowly return to the start position. After you complete the desired number of reps, repeat the process with your left arm.

Brad's Training Tips

- Don't twist your body to complete the move—this can result in injury.
- Keep your chin up at all times—this helps prevent rounding of the spine.

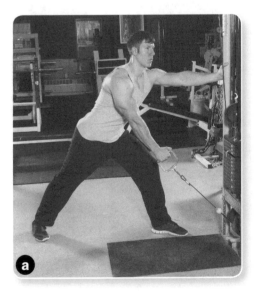

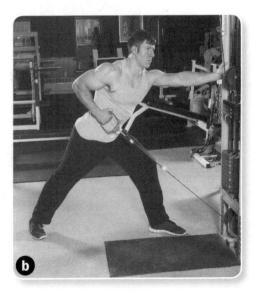

Chin-Up

Target

This move targets the back muscles. Secondary emphasis is on the biceps. This move is generally a bit easier to perform than the pull-up.

Start

Grasp a chinning bar with your hands approximately shoulder-width apart and your palms facing your body. Straighten your arms, bend your knees, and cross one foot over the other.

Movement

Keeping your upper body stable, pull your body up until your chin reaches the bar. Contract your lats. Return along the same path to the start position.

Brad's Training Tips

- Don't allow your body to swing—this introduces momentum into the movement, reducing tension to the target muscles.
- The chin-up can be very difficult to execute, especially for those who carry more weight in the lower body. If you can't reach your target rep range, consider using an assisted-chin device (such as a Gravitron) if your gym has one. Alternatively, enlist the help of a partner who can provide assistance by gently pulling up on your ankles as needed.

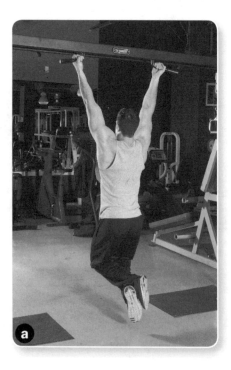 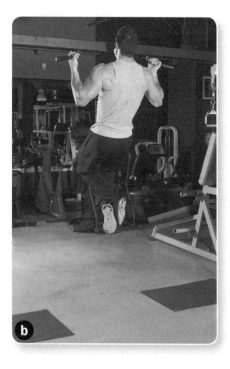

Pull-Up

Target

This move targets the back muscles.

Start

Grasp a chinning bar with your hands approximately shoulder-width apart and your palms facing away from your body. Straighten your arms, bend your knees, and cross one foot over the other.

Movement

Keeping your upper body stable, pull your body up until your chin reaches the bar. Contract your lats. Return along the same path to the start position.

Brad's Training Tips

- Don't allow your body to swing—this introduces momentum into the movement, reducing tension to the target muscles.

- The pull-up can be very difficult to execute, especially for those who carry more weight in the lower body. If you can't reach your target rep range, consider using an assisted-chin device (such as a Gravitron) if your gym has one. Alternatively, enlist the help of a partner who can provide assistance by gently pulling up on your ankles as needed.

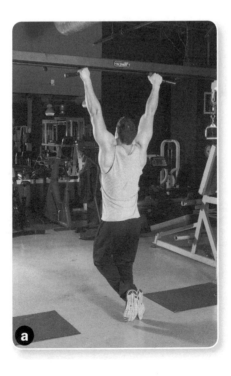
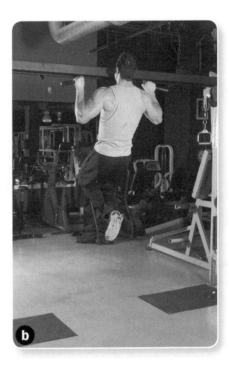

Lat Pull-Down

Target

This move targets the back muscles, particularly the lats.

Start

With your hands approximately shoulder-width apart and palms facing away from your body, grasp a lat pull-down bar attached to a lat pull-down machine. Secure your knees under the restraint pad and fully straighten your arms so that you feel a complete stretch in your lats. Tilt your body back slightly and keep your lower back arched throughout the move.

Movement

Pull the bar down to your upper chest, bringing your elbows back. Squeeze your shoulder blades together. Slowly reverse the direction and return to the start position.

Brad's Training Tips

- Don't lean back more than a few inches—doing so turns the move into a row rather than a pull-down.
- Don't swing your body as your perform the move—this introduces excessive momentum into the lift, reducing tension on the target muscles.

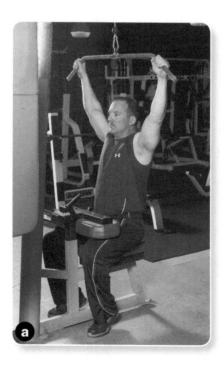

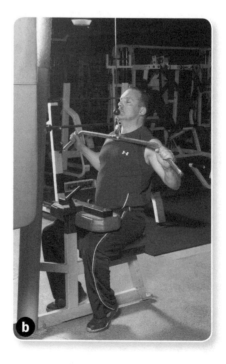

Neutral-Grip Lat Pull-Down

Target

This move targets the back muscles.

Start

Grasp a V-bar attached to a lat pull-down machine. Secure your knees under the restraint pad and fully straighten your arms so that you feel a complete stretch in your lats. Tilt your body back slightly and keep your lower back arched throughout the move.

Movement

Pull the bar to your upper chest, bringing your elbows back as you pull. Squeeze your shoulder blades together. Slowly reverse the direction and return to the start position.

Brad's Training Tips

- Don't lean back more than a few inches—doing so turns the move into a row rather than a pull-down.
- Don't swing your body as your perform the move—this introduces excessive momentum into the lift, reducing tension on the target muscles.

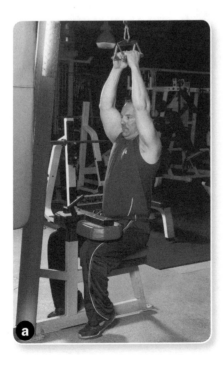
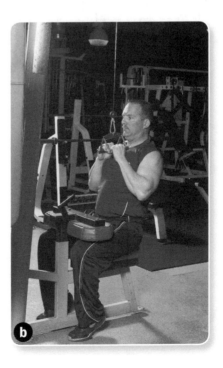

Reverse-Grip Lat Pull-Down

Target

This move targets the back muscles.

Start

Grasp a lat pull-down bar with your hands shoulder-width apart and your palms facing your body. Secure your knees under the restraint pad and fully straighten your arms so that you feel a complete stretch in your lats. Tilt your body back slightly and keep your lower back arched throughout the move.

Movement

Pull the bar to your upper chest, bringing your elbows back as you pull. Squeeze your shoulder blades together. Slowly reverse the direction and return to the start position.

Brad's Training Tips

- Don't lean back more than a few inches—doing so turns the move into a row rather than a pull-down.
- Don't swing your body as your perform the move—this introduces excessive momentum into the lift, reducing tension on the target muscles.

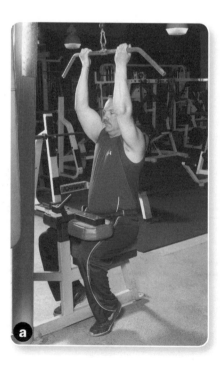
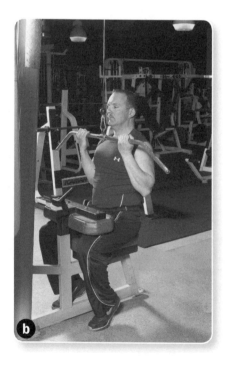

Cable Straight-Arm Lat Pull-Down

Target

This move targets the back muscles, particularly the lats.

Start

With your hands facing away from your body, grasp a straight bar attached to a high pulley. Slightly bend your elbows and bring the bar to eye level. Stand with your feet approximately shoulder-width apart. Slightly bend your knees and hold your core tight.

Movement

Keeping your upper body tilted forward slightly, pull the bar down until it touches your upper thighs. Contract your back muscles. Reverse the direction and slowly return to the start position.

Brad's Training Tip

■ You can perform this move with a variety of handle attachments, such as a rope, a curved bar, and loop handles.

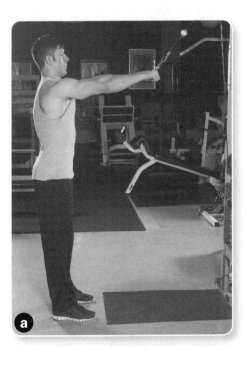 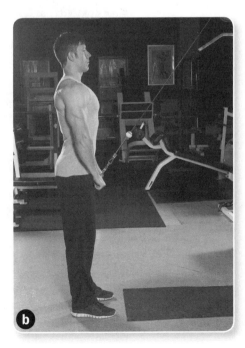

Cross Cable Lat Pull-Down

Target

This move targets the back muscles, particularly the lats.

Start

Grasp the loop handles of a high-pulley apparatus. Kneel on the floor facing away from the apparatus and fully extend your arms so that you feel a stretch in your lat muscles. Face your palms away from your body and slightly arch your lower back.

Movement

Keeping your body stable, pull the handles down and toward your sides, turning your palms in slightly on the descent. Contract your lats. Slowly reverse the direction and return to the start position.

Brad's Training Tip

- Don't allow your elbows to move forward during the move—this changes the plane of movement, altering muscle recruitment.

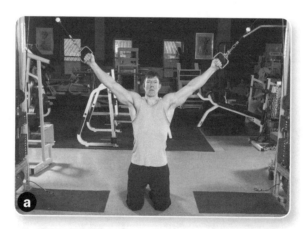

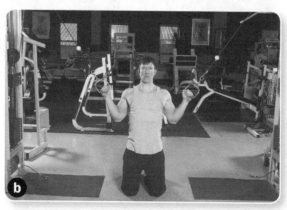

Dumbbell Incline Press

Target

This move targets the pectorals, particularly the upper part of the chest. It also significantly activates the triceps and front delts.

Start

Lie faceup on an incline bench and plant your feet firmly on the floor. Grasp two dumbbells with your palms facing away from your body. Bring the dumbbells to shoulder level so that they rest just above your armpits.

Movement

Simultaneously press both dumbbells directly over your chest, moving them in toward each other on the ascent. At the end of the movement, gently touch the sides of the dumbbells together. The weights should be over the upper portion of your chest. Contract your chest muscles. Slowly reverse the direction and return to the start position.

Brad's Training Tips

- Keep your elbows flared throughout the move—this helps maintain maximal activation of the pecs.
- As you press the weight, think of moving them in an inverted V pattern to increase range of motion.
- Your body should remain on the bench throughout the move and remain stable at all times.
- Don't lock your elbows at the end of the move—this prevents continuous muscle tension.

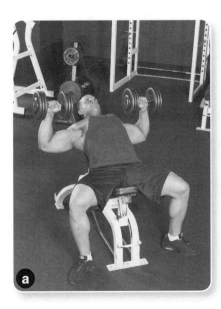

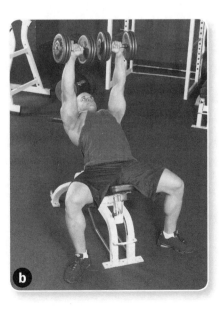

Dumbbell Decline Press

Target

This move targets the pectorals, particularly the lower fibers of the muscle. It also significantly activates the triceps.

Start

Lie faceup on a decline bench and secure your feet in the restraint pads. Grasp two dumbbells with your palms facing away from your body. Bring the dumbbells to shoulder level so that they rest just above your armpits.

Movement

Simultaneously press both dumbbells directly over your chest, moving them in toward each other on the ascent. At the end of the movement, gently touch the sides of the dumbbells together. The weights should be over the lower portion of your chest. Contract your chest muscles. Slowly reverse the direction and return to the start position.

Brad's Training Tips

■ Keep your elbows flared throughout the move—this maintains maximal activation of the pecs.

■ As you press the weight, think of moving them in an inverted V pattern to increase range of motion.

■ Your body should remain on the bench throughout the move and remain stable at all times.

■ Don't lock your elbows at the end of the move—this prevents continuous muscle tension.

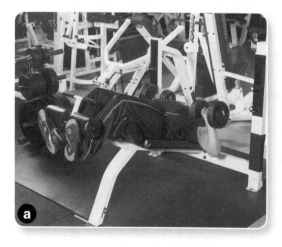
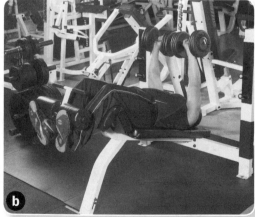

Dumbbell Chest Press

Target

This move targets the pectorals, particularly the sternal part of the chest.

Start

Lie faceup on a flat bench and plant your feet firmly on the floor. Grasp two dumbbells with your palms facing away from your body. Bring the dumbbells to shoulder level so that they rest just above your armpits.

Movement

Simultaneously press both dumbbells directly over your chest, moving them in toward each other on the ascent. At the end of the movement, gently touch the sides of the dumbbells together. The weights should be over the middle portion of your chest. Contract your chest muscles. Slowly reverse the direction and return to the start position.

Brad's Training Tips

- Keep your elbows flared throughout the move—this maintains maximal activation of the pecs.
- As you press the weight, think of moving them in an inverted V pattern to increase range of motion.
- Your body should remain on the bench throughout the move and remain stable at all times.
- Don't lock your elbows at the end of the move—this prevents continuous muscle tension.

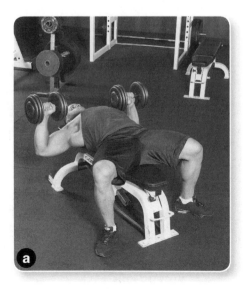 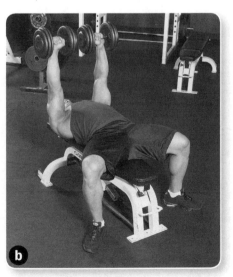

Barbell Incline Press

Target

This move targets the pectorals, particularly the upper part of the chest. It also significantly activates the triceps and front delts.

Start

Lie faceup on an incline bench set at approximately 30 to 40 degrees and plant your feet firmly on the floor. Grasp a barbell with your hands about shoulder-width apart and bring it down to the upper aspect of your chest.

Movement

Press the bar directly over your upper chest, moving it in a straight line into the air. At the end of the movement, the bar should be over the upper portion of your chest. Contract your chest muscles. Slowly return the bar along the same path to the start position.

Brad's Training Tips

- Keep your elbows flared throughout the move.
- Your body should remain on the bench throughout the move and remain stable at all times.
- Don't lock your elbows at the end of the move—this prevents continuous muscle tension.

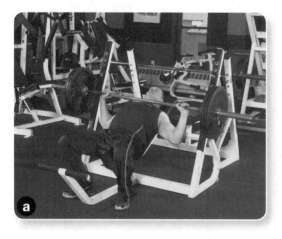
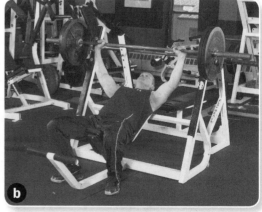

Barbell Chest Press

Target

This move targets the pectorals, particularly the sternal part of the chest. It also significantly works the triceps and front delts.

Start

Lie faceup on a flat bench and plant your feet firmly on the floor. Grasp a barbell with your hands approximately shoulder-width apart and bring it down to the middle of your chest.

Movement

Press the bar directly over your chest, moving it in a straight line into the air. At the end of the movement, the bar should be over the middle portion of your chest. Contract your chest muscles. Slowly return the bar along the same path to the start position.

Brad's Training Tips

- Keep your elbows flared throughout the move.
- Your body should remain on the bench throughout the move and remain stable at all times.
- To maintain continuous muscle tension, do not lock your elbows at the end of the move.

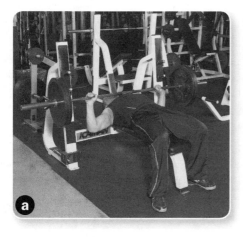
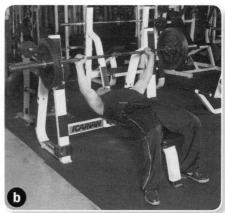

Barbell Decline Press

Target

This move targets the pectorals, particularly the lower part of the chest. It also significantly works the triceps and front delts.

Start

Lie faceup on a decline bench and secure your feet under the restraint pads. Grasp a barbell with your hands approximately shoulder-width apart and bring it down to the middle of your chest.

Movement

Press the bar directly over your chest, moving it in a straight line into the air. At the end of the movement, the bar should be over the lower portion of your chest. Contract your chest muscles. Slowly return the bar along the same path to the start position.

Brad's Training Tips

- Keep your elbows flared throughout the move.
- Your body should remain on the bench throughout the move and remain stable at all times.
- Don't lock your elbows at the end of the move—this prevents continuous muscle tension.

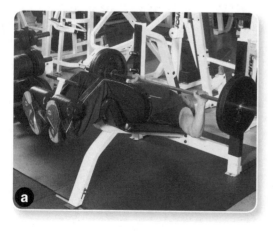
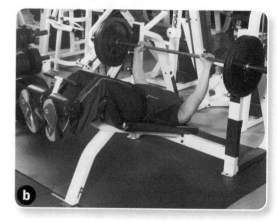

Machine Incline Press

Target

This move targets the pectorals, particularly the upper portion. Secondary emphasis is on the shoulders and triceps.

Start

Lie back on the seat of an incline press machine, set at approximately 40 degrees if it is adjustable, and align your upper chest with the handles on the machine. Grasp the handles with your hands shoulder-width apart and your palms facing away from your body. Flare your elbows.

Movement

Keeping your back against the support pad, press the handles forward, stopping just before you fully lock your elbows. Contract your chest muscles. Slowly reverse the direction and return to the start position.

Brad's Training Tips

- Depending on the machine, you may be able to adjust the incline of the bench to varying degrees to optimally target the upper chest in the incline press. Make sure that the action moves in line with the upper portion of your chest. A muscle always contracts maximally when the action is carried out in line with its fibers.

- Keep your elbows flared as you lift—allowing them to move forward changes the scope of the exercise.

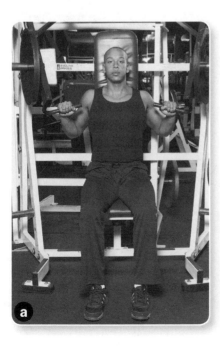
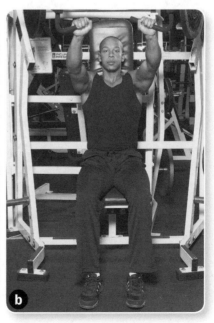

Machine Chest Press

Target

This move targets the chest muscles, particularly the sternal portion.

Start

Sit in a chest press machine and align your upper chest with the handles on the machine. Grasp the handles with your hands about shoulder-width apart and your palms facing away from your body.

Movement

Press the handles forward, stopping just before you fully lock out your elbows. Contract your chest muscles. Slowly reverse the direction and return to the start position.

Brad's Training Tip

- Keep your elbows flared as you lift so that they remain approximately parallel with the floor. Allowing them to move downward changes the plane of the exercise and alters muscle recruitment.

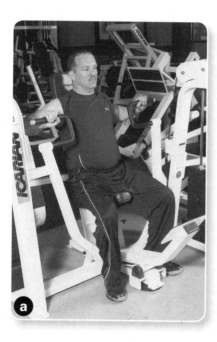

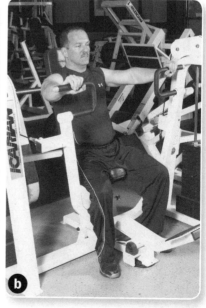

Dumbbell Flat Fly

Target

This move targets the pectorals, primarily the sternal fibers. It provides better isolation for the chest muscles than the flat press.

Start

Lie faceup on a flat bench and plant your feet firmly on the floor. Grasp two dumbbells and bring them out to your sides with a slight bend in your elbows. Face your palms in and toward the ceiling, and hold your upper arms roughly parallel with the level of the bench.

Movement

Raise the weights up in a semicircular motion and gently touch the weights together at the top of the move. At the end of the move, the dumbbells should be over the upper portion of your chest. Contract your chest muscles. Slowly return the weights along the same path to the start position.

Brad's Training Tips

- Keep your arms rounded throughout the move—do not straighten your elbows.
- As you lift the weights, think of hugging a beach ball.
- Your body should remain on the bench throughout the move and remain stable at all times.
- Avoid overstretching in the start position—this can cause injury.

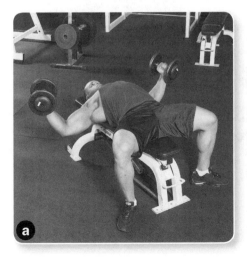 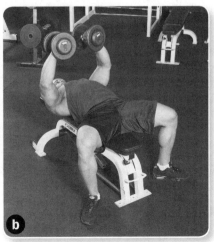

Dumbbell Incline Fly

Target

This move targets the pectorals, particularly the upper fibers. It provides better isolation for the chest muscles than the incline press.

Start

Lie faceup on an incline bench set at approximately 40 degrees and plant your feet firmly on the floor. Grasp two dumbbells and bring them out to your sides with a slight bend in your elbows. Face your palms in and toward the ceiling, and hold your upper arms roughly parallel with the level of the bench.

Movement

Slowly raise the weights upward in a circular motion and gently touch the weights together at the top of the move. At the end of the move, the dumbbells should be over the upper portion of your chest. Contract your chest muscles. Slowly return the weights along the same path to the start position.

Brad's Training Tips

- Keep your arms rounded throughout the move—do not straighten your elbows.
- As you lift the weights, think of hugging a beach ball.
- Your body should remain on the bench throughout the move and remain stable at all times.
- Avoid overstretching in the start position—this can cause injury.

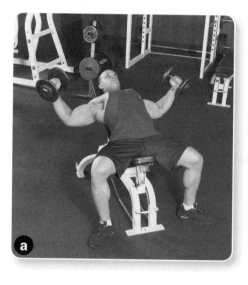
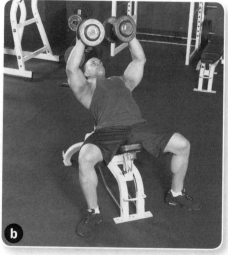

Pec Deck Fly

Target

This move targets the chest muscles.

Start

Grasp the handles of a pec deck machine with your palms facing away from your body. Slightly bend your elbows and keep your back immobile throughout the move.

Movement

Bring the handles together simultaneously and gently touch your hands together directly in front of your chest. Contract your pectoral muscles. Slowly reverse the direction and return to the start position.

Brad's Training Tip

- Several types of pec deck units exist. They all accomplish the same task, so use whatever version is available to you.

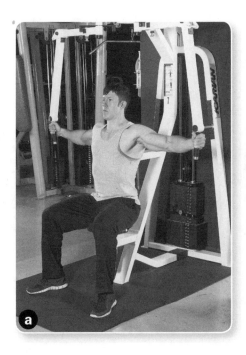
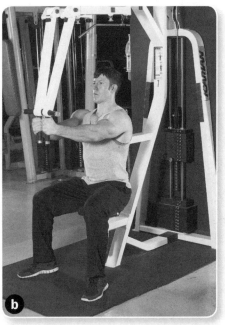

Cable Fly

Target

This move targets the chest muscles, particularly the sternal portion.

Start

Grasp the handles of a high-pulley apparatus. Stand with your feet about shoulder-width apart in a staggered stance and slightly bend your torso forward at the waist. Slightly bend your arms and hold them out to the sides so that they are approximately parallel with the floor.

Movement

Keeping your upper body motionless and your core tight, pull both handles down and across your body, creating a semicircular movement. Bring your hands together at the level of your waist and squeeze your chest muscles so that you feel a contraction in the midline area. Slowly reverse the direction and allow your hands to return along the same path to the start position.

Brad's Training Tip

■ Your elbows should remain slightly bent and fixed throughout the move—don't flex or extend them at any time. This error makes the exercise a pressing movement rather than a fly.

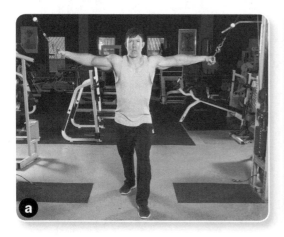
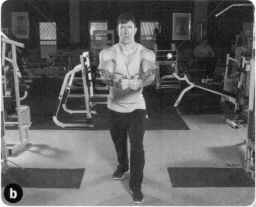

Chest Dip

Target

This move targets the pectorals, particularly the lower fibers.

Start

Place your hands on the parallel bars of a dip apparatus with your palms facing your sides. Hold your arms straight and slightly bend your knees and hips.

Movement

Leaning your torso forward, bend your arms and allow your elbows to flare out to the sides. Lower your body as far as comfortably possible. Feel a stretch in your pectoral muscles. Reverse the direction by straightening your arms until you reach the start position.

Brad's Training Tips

- If you cannot attain the necessary number of reps, enlist a partner to hold your feet and provide assistance. Alternatively, you can use an assisted-dip machine (such as the Gravitron).
- To increase the level of difficulty, place a dumbbell between your ankles.

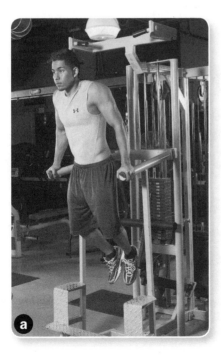
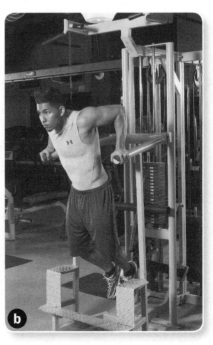

Crunch

Target

This move targets the abs, particularly the upper abdominal region.

Start

Lie faceup on the floor. Bend your knees and plant your feet. Press your lower back into the floor and fold your hands across your chest.

Movement

Keeping your lower back fixed to the floor, slowly raise your shoulders up and forward toward your chest. Contract your abdominal muscles. Slowly reverse the direction and return to the start position.

Brad's Training Tips

■ Don't allow your upper back touch the floor when lowering—doing so reduces tension to the abs.

■ If the move becomes easy, hold a weighted object such as a dumbbell or medicine ball against your chest.

■ Never place your hands behind your head—this facilitates pulling on the neck muscles, which can potentially lead to injury.

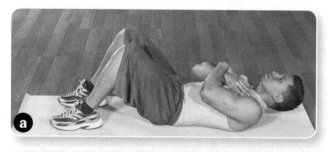

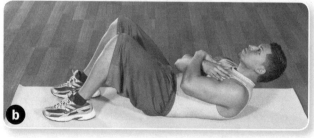

Reverse Crunch

Target

This move targets the abs, particularly the lower abdominal region.

Start

Lie faceup on the floor with your hands at your sides. Curl your knees into your abdomen and lift your butt so that it is slightly off the floor.

Movement

Keeping your upper back pressed into the floor, raise your butt as high as possible so that your pelvis tilts toward your chest. Contract your abs. Reverse the direction and return to the start position.

Brad's Training Tips

- Keep your upper torso completely stable—the only part of your body that should move is your hips and lumbar spine.
- Don't just push your butt up in the air. Rather, focus on pulling your pelvis toward your belly button. This forces the lower portion of the abs to do more of the work. It's a short range of motion that, when done properly, really hits the target muscle.
- Don't allow your butt to touch the floor when lowering—doing so reduces tension to the abs.
- If the move becomes easy, place a medicine ball between your thighs.

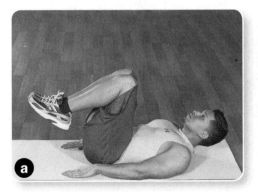
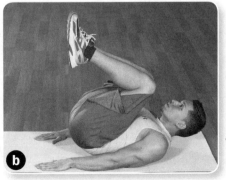

Bicycle Crunch

Target

This move targets the abs.

Start

Lie faceup on the floor and bend your legs about 40 degrees. Curl your hands and place them at your ears.

Movement

Slowly bring your left knee up toward your right elbow and try to touch them to one another. As you return your left leg and right elbow to the start position, bring your right leg toward your left elbow in the same manner. Continue this movement, alternating between right and left sides as if pedaling a bike.

Brad's Training Tips

- Never place your hands behind your head—this facilitates pulling on the neck muscles, which can potentially lead to injury.
- Avoid the temptation to speed up on this move. As with all exercise, perform in a smooth, controlled manner for optimal results.

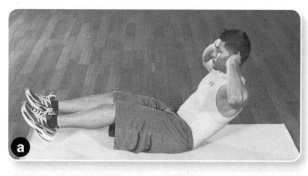

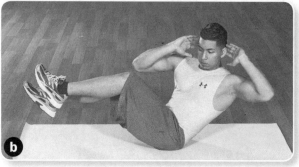

Roman Chair Side Crunch

Target

This move targets the obliques.

Start

Lie sideways on the top of a Roman chair with your feet secure under the restraint pads. Place your left fingertips by your left temple and your elbows wide of your body. Keep your bottom elbow flared with your hand on your hip.

Movement

Raise your top elbow so that your trunk laterally flexes as far as possible. Contract your obliques. Return along the same path to the start position. After you complete the desired number of reps, repeat the process on the opposite side.

Brad's Training Tip

- If you have trouble maintaining stability, hold onto the hip pad with your bottom hand.

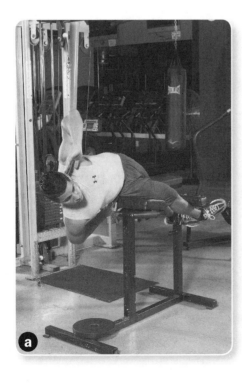
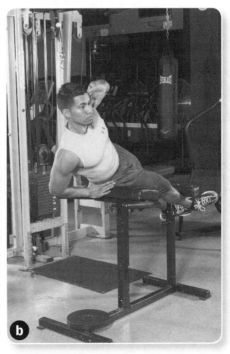

Stability Ball Abdominal Crunch

Target

This move targets the abs.

Start

Sit on top of a stability ball and place your feet shoulder-width apart. Walk your feet forward until the ball firmly supports your lower back. Place your hands on your chest and lower your upper back and shoulders onto the ball.

Movement

Lift your upper back and shoulders off the ball as far as comfortably possible. Contract your abs. Return along the same path to the start position.

Brad's Training Tips

- Sitting higher on the ball (i.e., butt on top of the ball) makes the exercise more difficult; sitting lower on the ball makes it easier.
- Keep your lower back on the ball at all times. Lifting your lower back engages the hip flexors, reducing stress to the target muscles.
- Keep your hips anchored so that you move over the ball and the ball does not roll under you.
- If the move becomes easy, hold a weighted object such as a dumbbell or medicine ball against your chest.

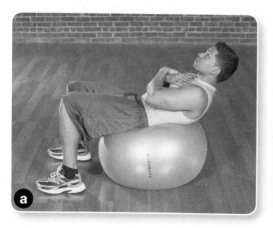
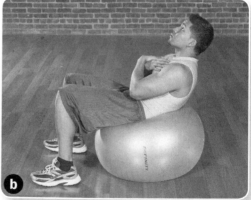

Cable Rope Kneeling Crunch

Target

This move targets the abs, particularly the upper portion.

Start

Face a high-pulley apparatus and kneel down to a seated position. Grasp the ends of a rope attached to the pulley. Place your elbows near your ears and hold your torso upright.

Movement

Keeping your lower back immobile, slowly curl your shoulders down, bringing your elbows down toward your knees. Contract your abs. Slowly uncurl your body and return to the start position.

Brad's Training Tip

- Curl only from your upper torso—your hips should remain fixed throughout the move. This maintains tension on the abs and removes activation of the hip flexors.

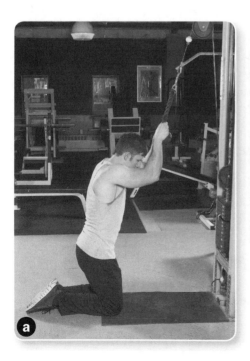
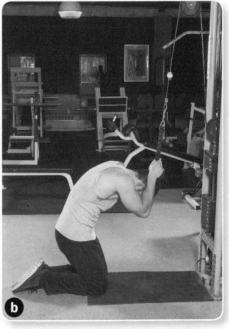

Cable Rope Kneeling Twisting Crunch

Target

This move targets the abs and obliques.

Start

Face a high-pulley apparatus and kneel down to a seated position. Grasp the ends of a rope attached to the pulley. Place your elbows near your ears and hold your torso upright.

Movement

Keeping your lower back immobile, slowly curl your shoulders down, twisting your body to the right as you bring your elbows toward your knees. Contract your abs. Slowly uncurl your body and return to the start position. Alternate twisting to the right and to the left for the desired number of reps.

Brad's Training Tip

■ Curl only from your upper torso—your hips should remain fixed throughout the move. This maintains tension on the target muscles and removes activation of the hip flexors.

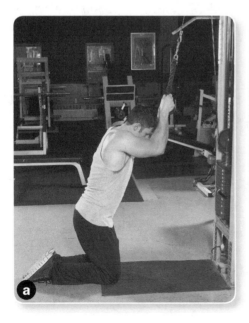
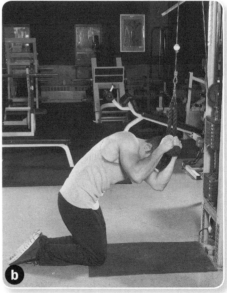

Toe Touch

Target

This move targets the abs, particularly the upper abdominal region.

Start

Lie faceup on the floor. Hold your arms and legs straight in the air, perpendicular to your body.

Movement

Keeping your lower back pressed to the floor, slowly curl your torso up and forward, moving your hands as close to your toes as possible. Contract your abs. Reverse the direction and return to the start position.

Brad's Training Tips

- Keep your lumbar region fixed throughout the move—only your upper back should rise off the floor.
- Keep your head stable at all times—any unwanted movement can potentially injure the cervical region.
- For added intensity, hold a weighted object such as a dumbbell or medicine ball in your hands.

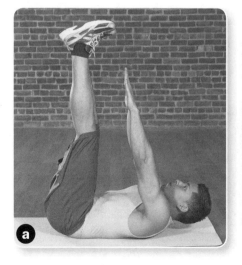
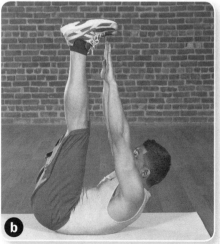

Plank

Target

This move targets the entire core.

Start

Lie facing down with your palms or forearms on the floor and your spine in a neutral position. Place your feet together.

Movement

Keeping your body as straight as possible, lift your body up, balancing your weight on your forearms and toes. Maintain this position for as long as possible. Return to the start position. Challenge yourself to maintain the plank position for longer periods of time.

Brad's Training Tips

- Use your core strength to keep your body rigid—don't allow any part of your body to sag at any time.
- Aim to work up to a hold of more than 60 seconds. Use a stopwatch to time yourself.
- To increase the level of difficulty, perform the move with one leg off the floor.
- For added intensity, perform the move on an unstable device such as a BOSU or a small stability ball.

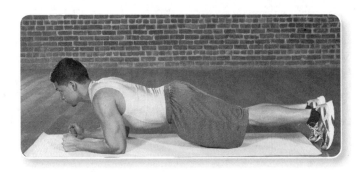

Side Bridge

Target

This move targets the entire core, particularly the obliques.

Start

Lie on your right side with your right forearm on the floor. Hold your legs straight and stack one foot on top of the other.

Movement

Straighten your right arm, keeping it in line with your shoulder, and place your left hand on your left hip so that your elbow is bent approximately 90 degrees. Hold this position for as long as possible. Repeat the process on the opposite side.

Brad's Training Tips

- Use your core strength to keep your body rigid—don't allow any part of your body to sag at any time.
- Balance on the sides of your foot, not the sole.
- Aim to work up to a hold of more than 60 seconds. Use a stopwatch to time yourself.
- To increase the level of difficulty, perform the move with your braced arm straight and your palm flat on the floor.
- For added intensity, perform the move on an unstable device such as a BOSU or a small stability ball.

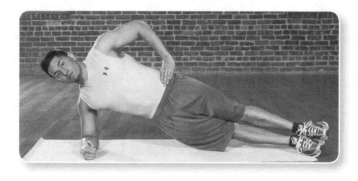

Hanging Knee Raise

Target

This move targets the abs.

Start

Grasp a chinning bar with your hands approximately shoulder-width apart and your palms facing away from your body. Bend your knees and stabilize your torso.

Movement

Keeping your knees bent, slowly raise your thighs upward, lifting your butt so that your pelvis tilts toward your abdomen. Contract your abs. Reverse the direction and return your legs to the start position. For increased intensity, straighten your legs while performing the move.

Brad's Training Tips

- Focus on pulling your pelvis up and back so that it approaches your belly button. This forces the lower portion of the abs to do more of the work.
- If you have trouble holding your body weight, consider using hanging ab straps.
- Keep your upper torso motionless throughout the move—don't swing to complete a repetition.

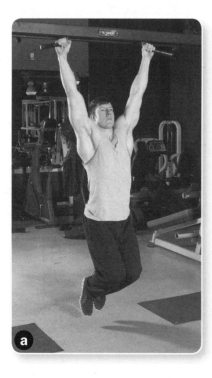 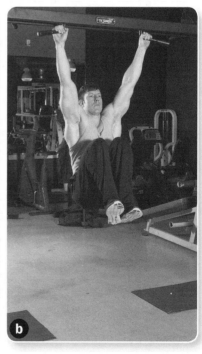

Russian Twist

Target

This move targets the obliques.

Start

Sit on the floor and rigidly hold your torso about 45 degrees to the floor. Grasp a medicine ball and hold it close to your torso. Bend your knees about 40 degrees and lift your feet slightly off the floor.

Movement

Keeping your lower body stable, twist your torso to one side as far as comfortably possible. Rotate back to center and repeat the process to the other side.

Brad's Training Tips

- Move only at the core—not at your shoulders or hips.
- Keep your eyes on your hands at all times to enhance core rotation.

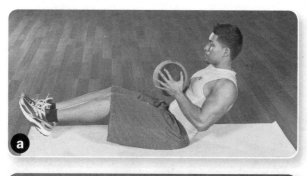

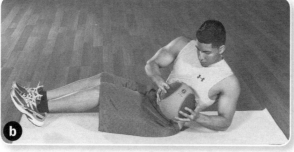

Dumbbell Side Bend

Target

This move targets the obliques.

Start

Grasp two dumbbells with your palms facing toward your body and allow them to hang at your sides. Stand with your feet about shoulder-width apart and slightly bend your knees.

Movement

Keeping your core tight, bend your torso to the left as far as comfortably possible. Contract your obliques. Return along the same path to the start position. Repeat on your right, then alternate sides until you complete the desired number of reps.

Brad's Training Tips

- The movement should take place solely at your waist—your hips shouldn't move at all during the move.
- Your upper body should remain upright at all times—don't sway forward or backward.

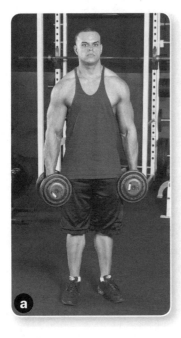 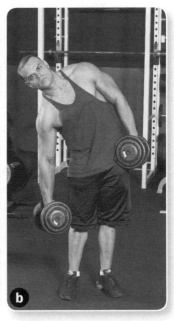

Cable Side Bend

Target

This move targets the obliques.

Start

With your left hand, grasp a loop handle attached to a low-pulley apparatus. Stand with your left side facing the machine and take a small step away from the unit so that there is tension in the cable. Keep your feet shoulder-width apart. Hold your torso erect and slightly bend your knees.

Movement

Keeping your core tight, bend your torso as far to the right as possible without discomfort. Contract your obliques. Return along the same path to the start position. After you complete the desired number of reps, repeat the process on the opposite side.

Brad's Training Tips

- The movement should take place solely at your waist—your hips shouldn't move at all during the move.
- Your upper body should remain in the same plane at all times—don't sway forward or backward.

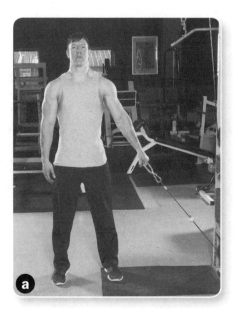
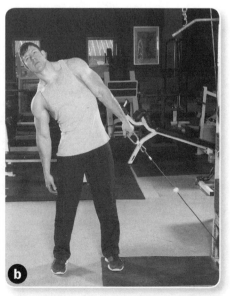

Cable Wood Chop

Target

This move targets the obliques.

Start

Grasp the ends of a rope attached to a cable-pulley apparatus. If possible, adjust the cable so that it is at chest height. (If the machine is not adjustable, you can perform the move from the high- or low-pulley positions.) Stand with your right side facing the machine and with your feet shoulder-width apart. Hold your torso erect and slightly bend your knees. Extend your arms across your body to the right as far as comfortably possible.

Movement

Keeping your lower body stable, pull the rope up and across your torso to the left (as if you were chopping wood). Contract your obliques. Return along the same path to the start position. After you complete the desired number of reps, repeat the process on the opposite side.

Brad's Training Tip

- To keep constant tension on the obliques, make sure the action takes place at your waist, not your hips.

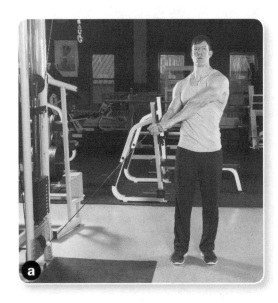
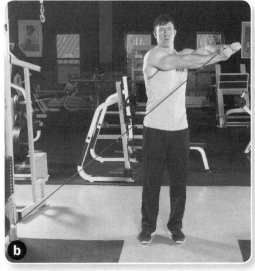

Barbell Rollout

Target

This move targets the abs.

Start

Load a pair of small plates (weights that are 5 pounds [2.3 kg] work well) onto the ends of a barbell. Grasp the middle of the bar with your hands approximately shoulder-width apart and your palms facing away from your body. Kneel down so that your shoulders are over the bar. Round your upper back and hold your butt up.

Movement

Keeping your knees fixed on the floor and your arms taut, roll the bar forward as far as comfortably possible without allowing your body to touch the floor. Reverse the direction by forcefully contracting your abs and return along the same path to the start position.

Brad's Training Tips

- To maximize activation of the abdominal musculature, the action should take place solely at the waist—not the hips.
- The contraction happens as you pull back to the start position—the rollout stretches the abs.

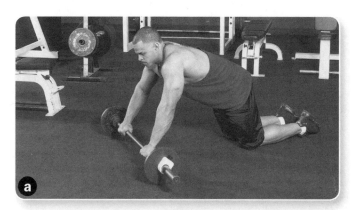

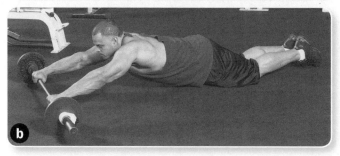

Exercises for the Shoulders and Arms

This chapter describes and illustrates exercises for the muscles of the shoulders and arms. Because these muscle groups reside on the extremities, they are generally more visible than the musculature of the torso and lower body. Hence, people tend to place increased emphasis on their development. Well-developed shoulders are essential for the classic v-taper look that delineates your silhouette. The biceps and triceps are the "show muscles" of the body. They epitomize strength and virility, accentuating the contours of your physique.

Read over the descriptions carefully and scrutinize the photos to ensure proper form. I provide training tips for each of these movements to optimize training performance. Remember that exercises are merely tools for achieving a means to an end—in this case, muscle development. If an exercise does not feel right to you, simply substitute a comparable move.

Arnold Press

Target

This move targets the deltoids. Secondary emphasis is on the upper trapezius and triceps.

Start

Sit at the edge of a flat bench. Grasp two dumbbells and bring the weights to shoulder level with your palms facing your body.

Movement

Press the dumbbells directly up and simultaneously rotate your hands so that your palms face forward during the last portion of the movement. Touch the weights together over your head. Slowly return the weights along the same arc, rotating your hands back to the start position.

Brad's Training Tip

- This shouldn't be a mechanical movement. Rotate your hands in a smooth motion as you press.

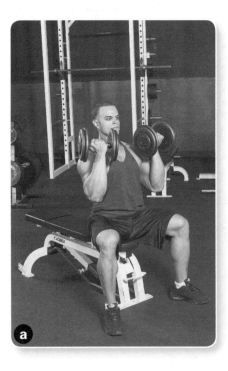
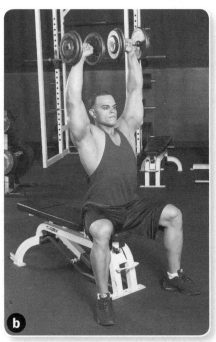

Military Press

Target

This move targets the shoulders, particularly the front delts. Secondary emphasis is on the upper trapezius and triceps.

Start

Assume a shoulder-width stance in front of a power rack. Grasp a barbell and bring it to the level of your upper chest with your palms facing away from your body.

Movement

Press the barbell directly up and over your head. Contract your deltoids at the top of the move. Reverse the direction and slowly return the bar along the same path to the start position.

Brad's Training Tips

- Keep your elbows forward, not flared, throughout the move to maintain movement in the sagittal plane.
- If you don't have access to a power rack, you will need to clean the bar to shoulder level.

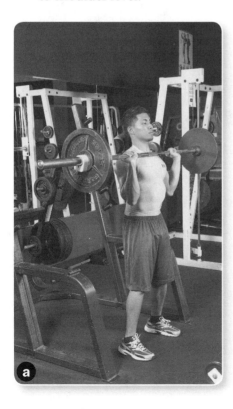
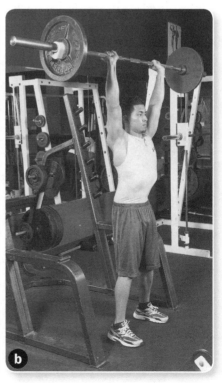

Dumbbell Shoulder Press

Target

This move targets the deltoids, particularly the front delts. Secondary emphasis is on the upper trapezius and triceps.

Start

Sit at the edge of a flat bench or chair. Grasp two dumbbells and bring the weights to shoulder level with your palms facing away from your body.

Movement

Press the dumbbells directly up and in. Touch the weights together directly over your head. Contract your deltoids. Slowly return the dumbbells along the same arc to the start position.

Brad's Training Tip

- Don't arc the weights outward as you press—this increases stress on the connective tissue in the shoulder joint.

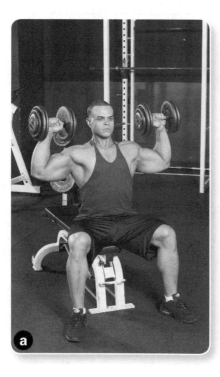
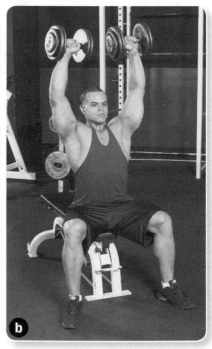

Machine Shoulder Press

Target

This move targets the deltoids, particularly the front delts. Secondary emphasis is on the upper trapezius and triceps.

Start

Sit upright in the seat of a shoulder-press machine and support your back on the pad. Grasp the handles of the machine with your palms facing away from your body and your elbows flared out to the sides. Adjust the seat height so that the handles are approximately in line with your shoulders.

Movement

Keeping your elbows flared, press the handles directly up and over your head. Contract your deltoids at the top of the move. Slowly return the handles to the start position.

Brad's Training Tips

- Don't lock your elbows at the top of the move—doing so reduces tension to the target muscles.
- Keep your elbows flared to the sides as you lift—allowing them to move forward changes the plane of the exercise.

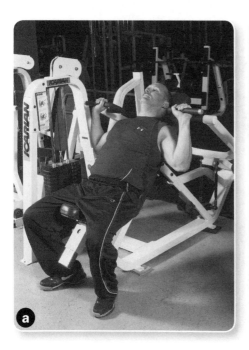 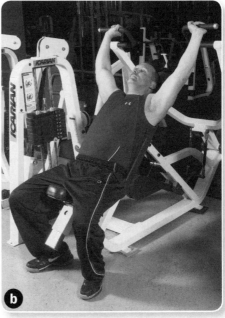

Dumbbell Lateral Raise

Target

This move targets the middle delts.

Start

Sit at the end of a flat bench with your back straight. Grasp two dumbbells and allow them to hang by your hips.

Movement

Keeping your elbows slightly bent, raise the dumbbells up and out to your sides until they reach shoulder level. At the top of the movement, the rear of the dumbbells should be slightly higher than the front. Contract your deltoids. Slowly return the weights along the same path to the start position.

Brad's Training Tips

- Think of pouring a cup of milk as you lift—this keeps maximum tension on the middle deltoids.
- You can also perform this move from a standing position.

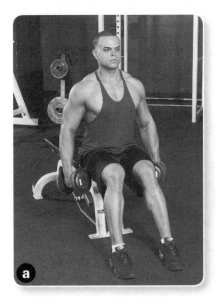 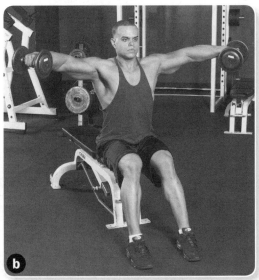

Machine Lateral Raise

Target

This move targets the middle delts.

Start

Sit in a lateral raise machine and press your torso to the chest pad. Adjust the seat so that your forearms align with the side pads. Place your forearms on the side pads and firmly grasp the attached handles with your palms facing each other.

Movement

Keeping your elbows flared, raise your upper arms up and out to the sides until they reach shoulder level. Contract your deltoids. Slowly return along the same path to the start position.

Brad's Training Tip

- Raise the weight only up to shoulder level—going higher than this can cause shoulder impingement.

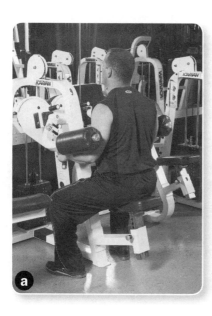
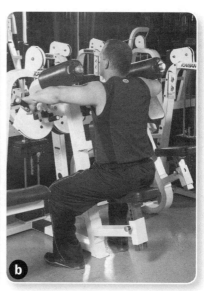

Cable Lateral Raise

Target

This move targets the middle delts.

Start

With your right hand, grasp a loop handle attached to a low-pulley apparatus. Face the pulley with your left side. Stand with your feet approximately shoulder-width apart and your torso erect. Slightly bend your knees and hold your core tight.

Movement

Maintain a slight bend to your elbow throughout the movement. Raise the handle across your body, up, and out to the side until it reaches the level of your shoulder. Contract your delts at the top of the movement. Slowly return the handle to the start position. After you complete the desired number of reps, repeat the process on your left side.

Brad's Training Tips

- Think of pouring a cup of milk as you lift. Your pinky should be slightly higher than your thumb at the top of the move—this keeps maximum tension on the middle deltoids.

- Keep your upper arms directly out to the sides at all times—allowing them to gravitate in switches the emphasis to the front delts at the expense of the middle delts.

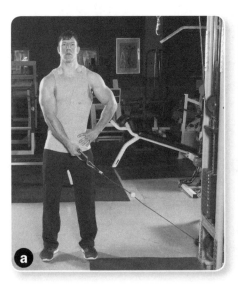

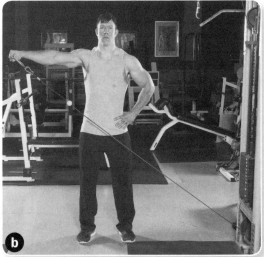

Dumbbell Bent Reverse Fly

Target

This move targets the posterior (rear) deltoid. I prefer this move to the standing version because it places less stress on the lower back.

Start

Grasp two dumbbells and sit at the edge of a bench or chair. Bend your torso forward so that it is almost parallel with the floor. Allow the dumbbells to hang down in front of your body.

Movement

Keeping your elbows slightly bent, raise the dumbbells up and out to your sides until they are parallel with the floor. Contract your delts at the top of the movement. Slowly return the dumbbells to the start position.

Brad's Training Tips

- Don't swing your body to complete a rep—this takes work away from the target muscles.
- Avoid the natural tendency to bring your elbows in toward the body as you lift. Hold your elbows out and away from the body throughout the move to keep tension on the rear delts.

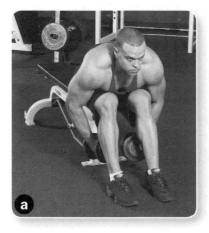
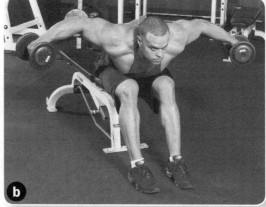

Machine Rear Delt Fly

Target

This move targets the posterior (rear) deltoid.

Start

Sit facing forward in a pec deck apparatus and press your chest up against the pad. Slightly bend your elbows and grasp the machine handles with your palms facing down.

Movement

Keeping your arms parallel with the floor, pull the handles back in a semicircular arc until they are approximately lateral with your torso. Contract your rear delts. Reverse the direction and return the handles to the start position.

Brad's Training Tip

- Keep your arms parallel with the floor throughout the move. If you are not able to keep your arms parallel, adjust the seat height accordingly.

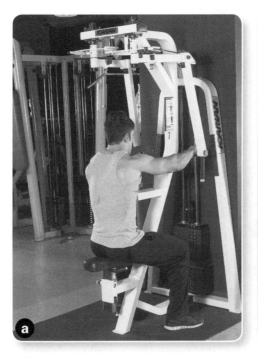

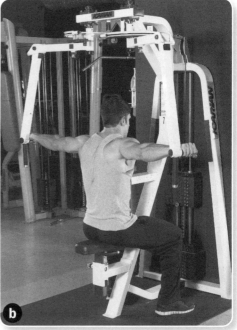

Cable Reverse Fly

Target

This move targets the posterior (rear) deltoid.

Start

Assume a shoulder-width stance in front of a cable pulley apparatus. Grasp the end of the left cable with your right hand and grasp the end of the right cable with your left hand. Keeping your torso rigid, take a couple steps back so that there is tension in the pulleys.

Movement

Keeping your arms slightly bent, simultaneously pull the cables out and back in a circular direction as far as comfortably possible. Contract your posterior deltoids. Return to the start position.

Brad's Training Tips

- Do not straighten your arms as you perform the move—this causes the triceps to assist in the movement.
- Don't swing your body to complete a rep—this takes work away from the target muscles.

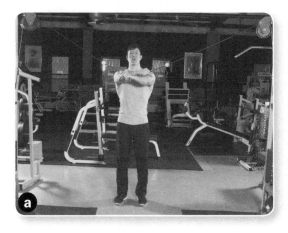
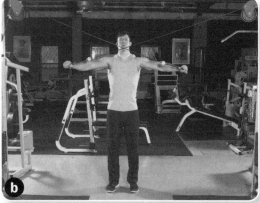

Cable Kneeling Reverse Fly

Target

This move targets the posterior (rear) deltoid.

Start

With your right hand, grasp a loop handle attached to the low-pulley apparatus of a cable apparatus. Kneel down on your hands and knees. Stabilize your torso with your left arm. Position your right arm by your side and slightly bend your right elbow.

Movement

Keep your elbow slightly bent and your core tight throughout the movement. Raise the handle out to your right side until your arm is parallel with the floor. Contract your delts at the top of the movement. Slowly return the handle to the start position. After you complete the desired number of reps, repeat the process on your left side.

Brad's Training Tip

■ Avoid the natural tendency to bring your elbows in toward your body as you lift. Hold your elbows away from your body throughout the movement to keep tension on the rear delts.

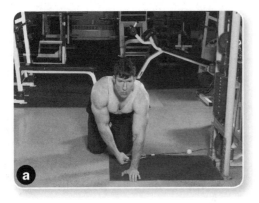
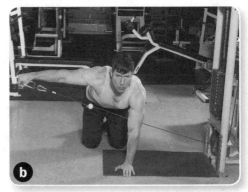

Barbell Upright Row

Target

This move targets the middle delts. Secondary emphasis is on the biceps.

Start

Grasp a barbell with a shoulder-width grip. Allow your arms to hang down from your shoulders with your palms facing your body. Assume a comfortable stance and bend your knees slightly.

Movement

Keeping your elbows higher than your wrists at all times, raise the bar up along the line of your body until your upper arms approach shoulder level. Contract your delts. Slowly lower the bar along the same path to the start position.

Brad's Training Tips

- Don't lift your elbows beyond a position that is parallel with the floor. Doing so can lead to shoulder impingement, which injures the rotator cuff.
- Keep the bar as close to your body as possible throughout the movement.

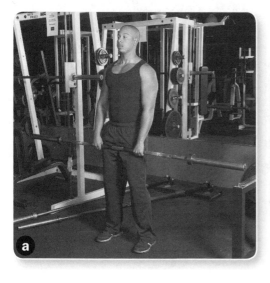
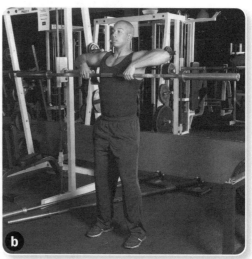

Cable Upright Row

Target

This move targets the middle delts. Secondary emphasis is on the biceps.

Start

Grasp the ends of a rope (or the loop handles) attached to a low-pulley apparatus. Stand with your feet shoulder-width apart and your torso erect. Slightly bend your knees and hold your core tight. Allow your arms to hang down from your shoulders in front of your body, but don't lock your elbows.

Movement

Pull the rope up along the line of your body until your upper arms approach shoulder level. Keep your elbows higher than your wrists at all times. Contract your delts. Slowly lower the rope along the same path to the start position.

Brad's Training Tips

- Initiate the action by lifting the elbows, not the wrists, to ensure optimal stimulation of the target muscles.
- Don't lift your elbows beyond a position that is parallel with the floor. Doing so can lead to shoulder impingement, which injures the rotator cuff.
- Keep your hands as close to your body as possible throughout the entire move.
- Perform the move with a straight bar if you desire.

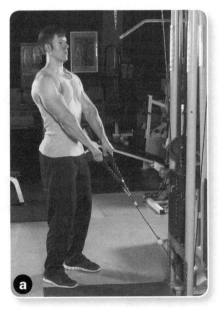 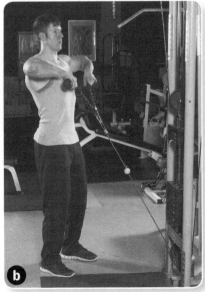

Dumbbell Standing Biceps Curl

Target

This move targets the biceps.

Start

Assume a shoulder-width stance and slightly bend your knees. Grasp a pair of dumbbells and allow them to hang at your sides with your palms facing forward.

Movement

Press your elbows into your sides and keep them stable throughout the move. Curl the dumbbells up toward your shoulders. Contract your biceps at the top of the move. Slowly reverse the direction and return to the start position.

Brad's Training Tips

- If desired, begin with your palms facing your sides and actively supinate your hands as you lift.
- Keep your wrists straight as you lift—don't roll them to complete the move.
- You can also perform this move from a seated position.

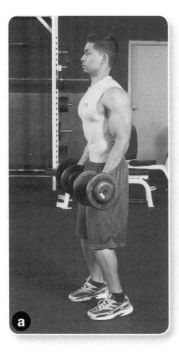 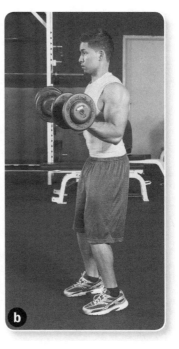

Dumbbell Incline Biceps Curl

Target

This move targets the biceps. Because the arms are kept back, this move is especially effective for targeting the long head.

Start

Lie faceup on an incline bench set at 40 degrees. Grasp two dumbbells and allow the weights to hang behind your body with your palms facing forward.

Movement

Keeping your upper arms stable, curl the dumbbells up toward your shoulders. Contract your biceps. Slowly return the weights to the start position.

Brad's Training Tips

- Keep your elbows back throughout the movement—this keeps maximal tension on the biceps, especially the long head.
- Keep your wrists straight as you lift—don't roll them to complete the move.

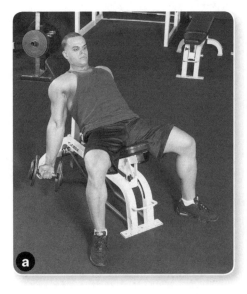
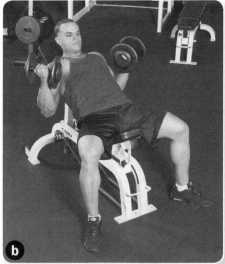

Dumbbell Facedown Incline Curl

Target

This move targets the biceps. Because the arms are held in front of the body, this move is especially effective for targeting the short head.

Start

Lie facedown on an incline bench set at 30 degrees. Grasp two dumbbells and allow the weights to hang straight down from your shoulders with your palms facing away from your body.

Movement

Keeping your upper arms stable throughout the movement, curl the dumbbells up toward your shoulders. Contract your biceps. Slowly return the weights to the start position.

Brad's Training Tips

- Don't swing your arms as you lift—this introduces momentum into the movement and reduces stress to the target muscles.
- Keep your wrists straight as you lift—don't roll them to complete the move.

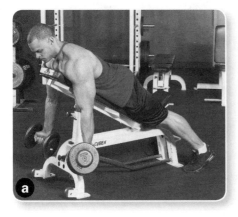
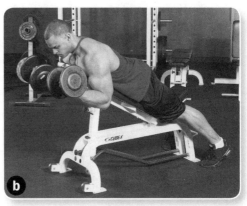

Dumbbell Preacher Curl

Target

This move targets the biceps, particularly the short head.

Start

Grasp a dumbbell with your left hand. Place the upper portion of your left arm on a preacher curl bench and extend your left forearm just short of locking out the elbow.

Movement

Keeping your upper arm pressed to the bench, curl the dumbbell up toward your shoulder. Contract your biceps. Slowly return the weight to the start position. After you complete the desired number of reps, repeat the process on your right side.

Brad's Training Tips

- Fully brace your upper arm on the bench—there should be no space between your arm and the bench.
- Keep your wrists straight as you lift—don't roll them to complete the move.
- If you do not have access to a preacher curl bench, use an incline bench instead.

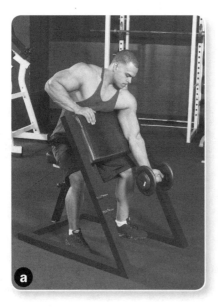 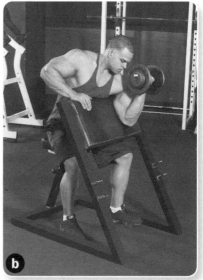

Barbell Preacher Curl

Target

This move targets the biceps, particularly the short head.

Start

Grasp a barbell with both hands. Place the upper portion of your arms on a preacher curl bench and extend your forearms just short of locking out the elbow.

Movement

Keeping your upper arms pressed to the bench, curl the bar up toward your shoulders. Contract your biceps. Slowly return the bar to the start position.

Brad's Training Tips

- Fully brace your upper arms on the bench—there should be no space between your arms and the bench.
- Keep your wrists straight as you lift—don't roll them to complete the move.

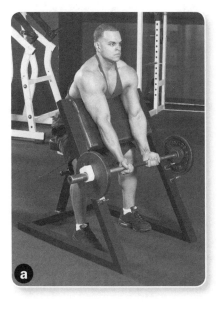 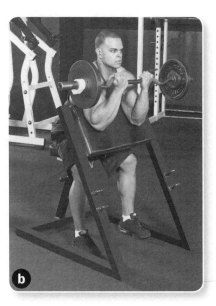

Machine Preacher Curl

Target

This move targets the biceps, particularly the short head.

Start

Sit upright in a curl machine. Adjust the seat so that your armpits align with the top of the pad. Grasp the machine handles with your palms facing your body and place the back of your arms on the pad.

Movement

Keeping your torso erect, raise the handles toward your shoulders as far as comfortably possible. Contract your biceps. Reverse the direction and return to the start position.

Brad's Training Tip

- To maintain optimal tension on the biceps, press your upper arms to the pads throughout the entire movement.

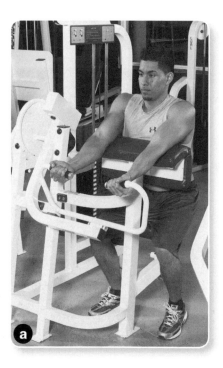 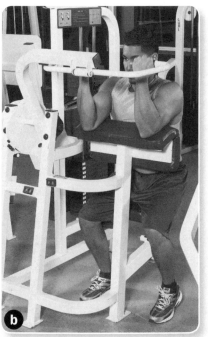

Concentration Curl

Target

This move targets the biceps, particularly the short head.

Start

Sit at the edge of a flat bench with your legs wide apart. Grasp a dumbbell in your right hand and brace your right triceps on the inside of your right thigh. Straighten your arm so that it hangs down near the floor.

Movement

Curl the weight up and in along the line of your body. Contract your biceps at the top of the move. Reverse the direction and slowly return to the start position. After you complete the desired number of reps, repeat the process on your left side.

Brad's Training Tips

- Brace your exercising arm on your inner thigh at all times. If you struggle to complete a rep, use your opposite hand to assist the move—don't swing your exercising arm.
- Keep your wrists straight as you lift—don't roll them to complete the move.

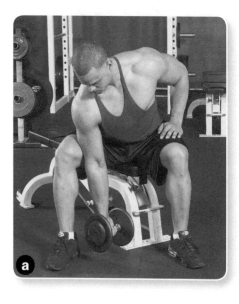 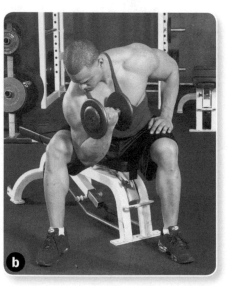

Dumbbell Standing Hammer Curl

Target

This move targets the upper arms, particularly the brachialis.

Start

Assume a shoulder-width stance and slightly bend your knees. Grasp a pair of dumbbells and allow them to hang at your sides with your palms facing each other.

Movement

Keeping your elbows pressed into your sides, curl the dumbbells up toward your shoulders. Contract your biceps at the top of the move. Slowly reverse the direction and return to the start position.

Brad's Training Tip

■ Keep your wrists straight as you lift—don't roll them to complete the move.

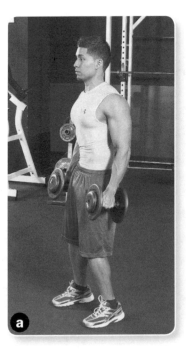 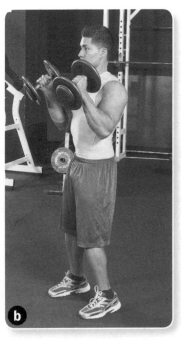

Barbell Curl

Target

This move targets the biceps.

Start

Assume a comfortable stance and bend your knees slightly. Grasp a barbell with a shoulder-width grip with your palms facing up.

Movement

Keeping your upper arms pressed into your sides, curl the bar up toward your shoulders. Contract your biceps at the top of the move. Slowly reverse the direction and return to the start position.

Brad's Training Tips

- Keep your upper arms motionless throughout the move—all activity takes place at the elbow
- You can perform this move with either a straight bar or an EZ-curl bar. The EZ-curl bar can help alleviate pressure on your wrists.

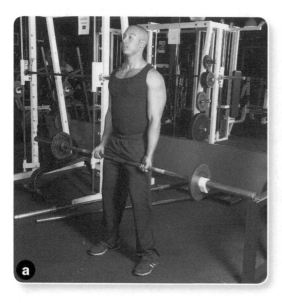
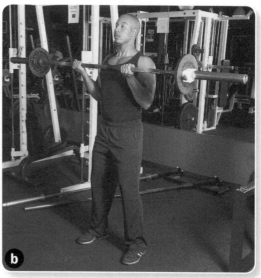

Barbell Drag Curl

Target

This move targets the biceps, particularly the long head.

Start

Grasp a barbell with a shoulder-width grip with your palms facing up. Allow the bar to hang in front of your body and slightly bend your elbows. Assume a comfortable stance and slightly bend your knees.

Movement

Keeping your upper arms close to your sides and stable throughout the move, bring your elbows behind your body, curling the bar along the line of your torso up toward your shoulders. Contract your biceps. Slowly reverse the direction and return to the start position.

Brad's Training Tip

- Move your elbows back as you lift—this keeps maximum tension on the long head.

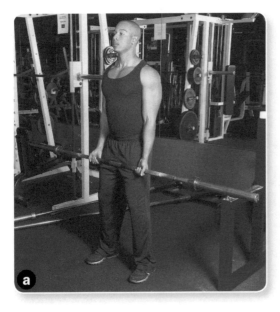
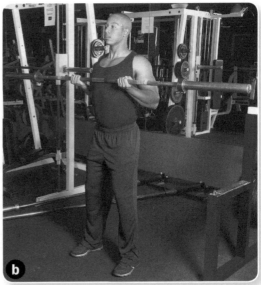

Cable Rope Hammer Curl

Target

This move targets the upper arms, particularly the brachialis.

Start

Grasp both ends of a rope (or loop handles) attached to a low-pulley apparatus. Press your elbows into your sides with your palms facing each other. Stand with your feet shoulder-width apart and your torso erect. Slightly bend your knees and hold your core tight.

Movement

Keeping your arms stable throughout the move, curl the rope up toward your shoulders. Contract your biceps at the top of the move. Slowly reverse the direction and return to the start position.

Brad's Training Tips

- Don't allow your upper arm to move forward as you lift—this brings your shoulders into the movement at the expense of your arm muscles.
- Keep your wrists straight as you lift—don't roll them to complete the move.

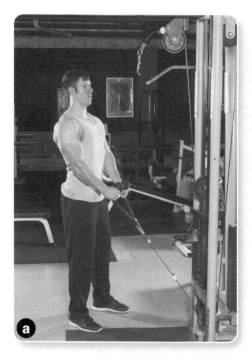 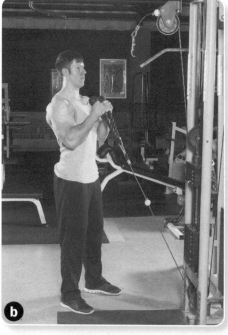

Cable Curl

Target

This move targets the biceps.

Start

Grasp a straight bar attached to a low-pulley apparatus. Press your elbows into your sides with your palms facing up. Stand with your feet shoulder-width apart and your torso erect. Slightly bend your knees and hold your core tight.

Movement

Keeping your upper arms stable throughout the move, curl the bar up toward your shoulders. Contract your biceps. Slowly reverse the direction and return to the start position.

Brad's Training Tips

- Keep your wrists straight as you lift—don't roll them.
- Don't allow your upper arm to move forward as you lift—this brings your shoulders into the movement at the expense of your arm muscles.

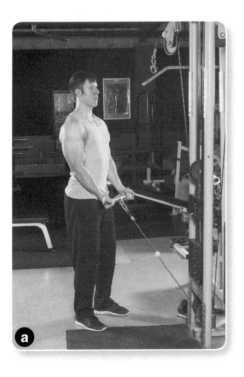

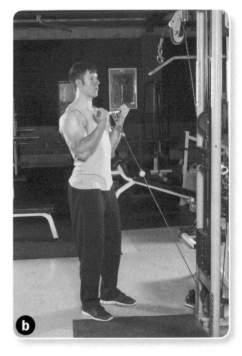

Cable One-Arm Curl

Target

This move targets the biceps.

Start

With your right hand, grasp a loop handle attached to a low-pulley apparatus. Press your right elbow into your right side. Stand with your feet shoulder-width apart and your torso erect. Slightly bend your knees and hold your core tight.

Movement

Keeping your upper arm stable throughout the move and your palm facing up, curl the handle up toward your shoulder. Contract your biceps. Slowly reverse the direction and return to the start position. After you complete the required number of reps, repeat the process on your left side.

Brad's Training Tips

- Keep your wrists straight as you lift—don't roll them.
- Don't allow your upper arm to move forward as you lift—this brings your shoulders into the movement at the expense of your arm muscles.

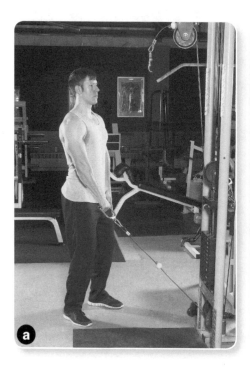

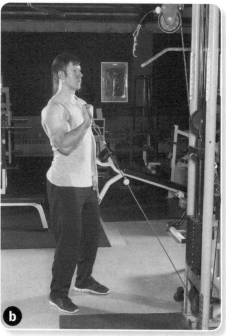

Dumbbell Overhead Triceps Extension

Target

This move targets the triceps, particularly the long head.

Start

Grasp the stem of a dumbbell with both hands. Sit at the edge of a flat bench or chair and bring the dumbbell overhead. Bend your elbows and allow the weight to hang down behind your head as far as comfortably possible.

Movement

Keeping your elbows back and pointed toward the ceiling, straighten your arms. Contract your triceps. Reverse the direction and slowly lower the weight along the same path to the start position.

Brad's Training Tips

- Keep your elbows pinned to your ears as you lift—if your elbows flare, you'll reduce stress to the triceps.
- If you have difficulty maintaining erect posture, place the bench in an upright position and brace your back against the pad.
- If desired, perform this exercise with one arm at a time. This may help alleviate stress on the elbow and allow you to focus on each arm individually.

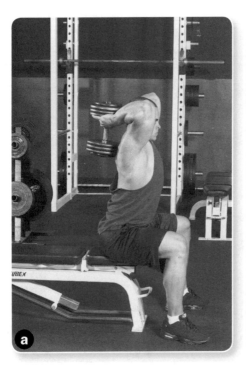
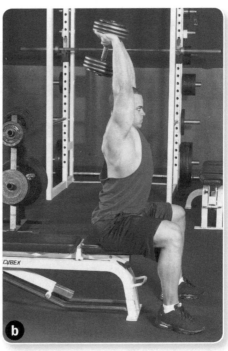

Cable Rope Overhead Triceps Extension

Target

This move targets the triceps, particularly the long head.

Start

Grasp the ends of a rope (or loop handles) attached to a high-pulley apparatus and turn your body away from the weight stack. Press your elbows close to your ears and bend your elbows. Allow your hands to hang behind your head with your palms facing each other as far as comfortably possible. Bring one foot in front of the other. Stand with your torso erect and bend your knees slightly.

Movement

Keeping your elbows close to your ears, straighten your arms as fully as possible. Contract your triceps. Reverse the direction and slowly return the weight along the same path to the start position.

Brad's Training Tips

- Pin your elbows to your ears as you lift—if your elbows flare, you'll reduce stress to the triceps.
- Keep your upper arms completely stationary throughout the move—any forward movement diminishes tension on the triceps.
- If you desire, perform this exercise with one arm at a time. This may alleviate stress on the elbow and allow you to focus on each arm individually.

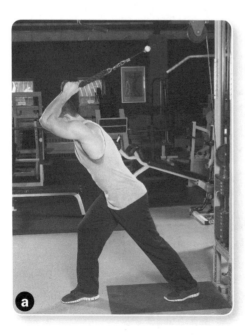 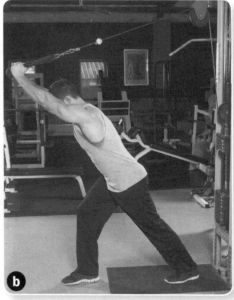

Nosebreaker

Target

This move targets the triceps.

Start

Lie faceup on a flat bench and plant your feet firmly on the floor. Grasp a barbell and straighten your arms so that the barbell is directly over your chest. Your arms should be perpendicular to your body.

Movement

Keeping your elbows in and pointed toward the ceiling, slowly lower the dumbbells until they reach a point just above the level of your forehead. Reverse the direction and press the dumbbells up until they reach the start position.

Brad's Training Tips

- Pin your elbows to your ears as you lift—if your elbows flare, you'll reduce stress to the triceps.
- You can perform this exercise with one arm at a time with a dumbbell. This allows you to focus on each arm individually.

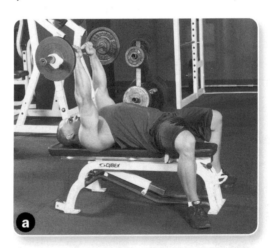

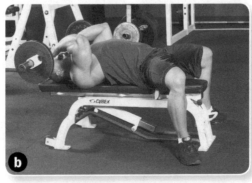

Machine Nosebreaker

Target

This move targets the triceps

Start

Sit in the machine and align the seat so that your upper arms rest comfortably on the pad and are approximately parallel with the ground. Grasp the handles of the machine with your palms facing one another.

Movement

Keeping your torso erect and elbows in, push the handles down until your arms fully straighten. Contract your triceps. Reverse the direction and return to the start position.

Brad's Training Tip

- Keep your upper arms in contact with the pad at all times throughout the move. Otherwise, secondary muscles will take over the exercise.

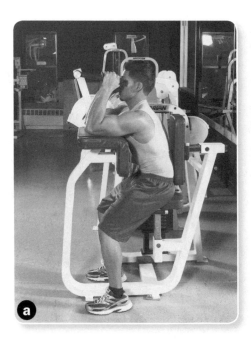
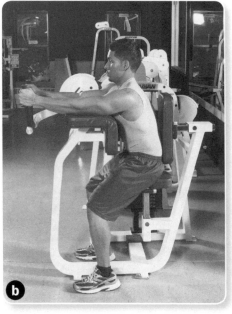

Dumbbell Triceps Kickback

Target

This move targets triceps, particularly the middle and lateral heads.

Start

Stand with your body bent forward so that it is almost parallel with the floor. Grasp a dumbbell with your left hand and press your left arm against your side. Bend your elbows 90 degrees.

Movement

With your palm facing your body, straighten your arm until it is parallel with the floor. Reverse the direction and return the weight to the start position. After you complete the desired number of reps, repeat the process on your right side.

Brad's Training Tips

- Don't let your upper arm sag down as you lift—this reduces the effects of gravity and thus diminishes tension to the target muscles.
- Don't flick your wrists at the top of the movement—this common error fatigues the forearm muscles before the triceps and reduces the effectiveness of the move.

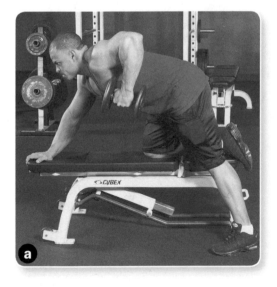
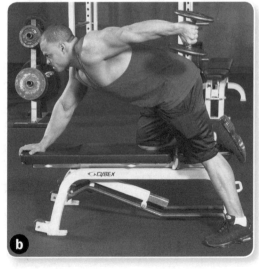

Cable Triceps Kickback

Target

This move targets the triceps, particularly the middle and lateral heads.

Start

Grasp a loop handle attached to a low-pulley apparatus. Bend your torso forward so that it is roughly parallel with the floor. Press your right arm against your side with your palm facing back. Bend your right elbow 90 degrees. Stand with your feet approximately shoulder-width apart in a staggered stance and your back straight. Bend your knees slightly and hold onto a sturdy part of the machine with your left hand for support.

Movement

Keeping your upper arm stable, straighten your arm until it is parallel with the floor. Reverse the direction and return the weight to the start position. After you complete the desired number of reps, repeat the process on your left side.

Brad's Training Tips

- Don't let your upper arm sag as you lift—this reduces the effects of gravity and thus diminishes tension to the target muscles.
- Don't flick your wrists at the top of the movement—this common error fatigues the forearm muscles before the triceps and reduces the effectiveness of the move.
- Arch your back slightly throughout the movement. Never round your spine—this places stress on the lumbar area and could lead to injury.

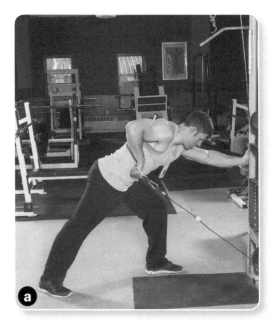
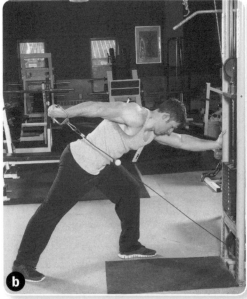

Bench Press

Target

This move targets the triceps. It also works the pecs significantly.

Start

Lie faceup on a flat bench and plant your feet firmly on the floor. Grasp a barbell with your hands approximately 1 foot (0.3 m) apart. Bring the bar directly under your pecs.

Movement

Keeping your elbows close to your sides, press the weight straight up over your chest. Contract your triceps. Slowly return the bar along the same path to the start position.

Brad's Training Tip

■ Don't grip the bar with your hands too close together—this causes the elbows to flare, reducing stress to the triceps.

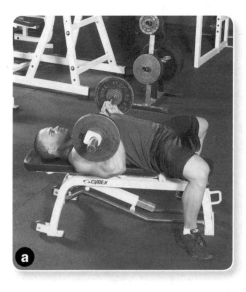

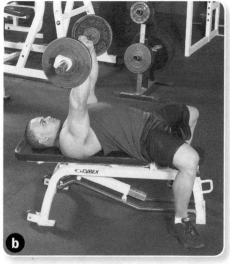

Cable Triceps Press-Down

Target

This move targets the triceps, particularly the middle and lateral heads.

Start

With your palms facing away from your body, grasp the ends of a rope (or loop handles) attached to a high-pulley apparatus. Stand with your feet shoulder-width apart and your torso erect. Slightly bend your knees and hold your core tight. Bend your elbows 90 degrees. Press your arms against your sides with your palms facing each other.

Movement

Keeping your elbows at your sides, straighten your arms as far as possible without discomfort. Contract your triceps. Reverse the direction and return to the start position.

Brad's Training Tips

- Don't allow your arms to move out as you lift—this brings the chest muscles into play at the expense of your triceps.
- For an added contraction, turn your palms out so that they face away from each other at the end of the move.
- You can perform this move with a variety of attachments, including a curved bar, a straight bar, and loop handles.

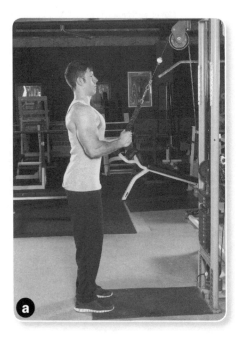 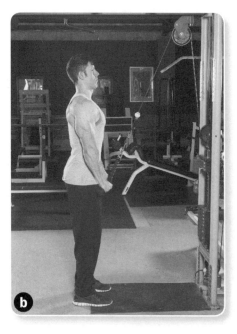

Triceps Dip

Target

This move targets the triceps.

Start

Set up two flat benches several feet apart so that they are parallel with each other. Hold your arms straight and place your palms on the edge of one bench. Place your heels on top of the other bench.

Movement

Slowly bend your elbows as far as comfortably possible and allow your butt to descend below the level of the bench. Make sure that your elbows stay close to your body throughout the move. Reverse the direction by forcibly straightening your arms and return to the start position.

Brad's Training Tips

- Make the move easier by placing your feet on the floor.
- Increase the intensity of the exercise by placing a weight plate on your lap (variation photo).
- Keep your back close to the bench at all times. If your body gravitates forward, you place increased stress on the shoulder joint.

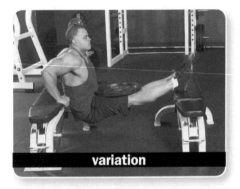

variation

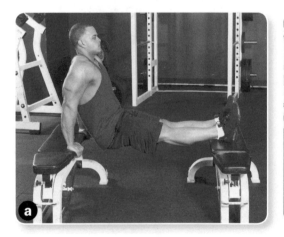

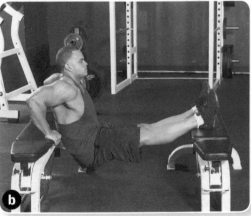

Machine Triceps Dip

Target

This move targets the triceps.

Start

Sit upright in the seat of a triceps dip machine and secure your knees firmly under the pads. Grasp the machine handles with your palms facing your sides so that your arms form an angle of approximately 90 degrees.

Movement

Keeping your torso erect and elbows in, push the handles down until your arms fully straighten. Contract your triceps. Reverse the direction and return to the start position.

Brad's Training Tip

■ Keep your upper arms close to your body at all times. Allowing the elbows to flare increases pectoral activation and thereby reduces the work performed by the triceps.

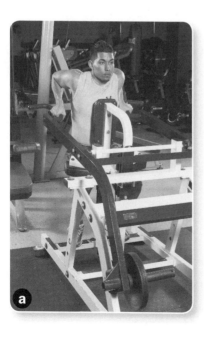
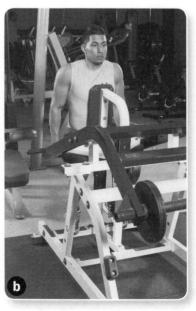

CHAPTER 5

Exercises for the Lower Body

This chapter describes and illustrates exercises for the muscles of the lower body: the quadriceps, gluteals, hamstrings, and calves. Despite their functional and aesthetic importance, a majority of guys seem to train these muscles as an afterthought, performing a few half-hearted sets with minimal effort. Some misguided souls choose to neglect working the leg muscles altogether, figuring if they simply wear pants all the time then no one will notice. Big mistake. Not only are strong, powerful looking legs an essential part of a balanced physique (face it, you look pretty silly wearing long pants to the beach or a pool party!), but lower-body training can actually have an anabolic effect on the entire body, helping to spur overall growth and thus maximize your muscular potential. Bottom line: Train your legs and train them hard!

Read over the descriptions carefully and scrutinize the photos to ensure proper form. I provide training tips for each of these movements to optimize training performance. Remember that exercises are merely tools for achieving a means to an end—in this case, muscle development. If an exercise does not feel right to you, simply substitute a comparable move.

Walking Lunge

Target

This move targets the quads and glutes. Secondary emphasis is on the hamstrings.

Start

Grasp two dumbbells. Stand in an open area with your feet shoulder-width apart.

Movement

Take a long stride forward with your right leg and bring your left knee to just above floor level. Then, keeping your shoulders back and your head up throughout the move, step forward with your left leg and allow your right knee to drop down until it is a few inches (about 10 cm) from the floor. Alternate legs and continue for the desired number of reps.

Brad's Training Tip

■ Do not push forward with your front leg—doing so can place undue stress on the knee. Rather, focus on passively dropping the rear leg so that the front leg forms a 90-degree angle in the bottom position.

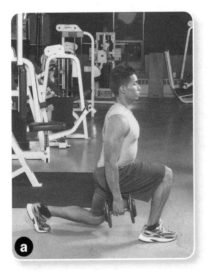 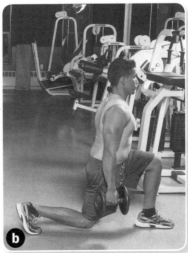

Barbell Lunge

Target

This move targets the quads and glutes. Secondary emphasis is on the hamstrings.

Start

Rest a barbell across your shoulders, grasping the bar on both sides to maintain balance. Assume a shoulder-width stance and hold your shoulders back and your chin up.

Movement

Keeping your core tight, take a long step forward with your left leg, slowly lowering your body by flexing your left knee and hip in the process. Continue your descent until your right knee is almost in contact with the floor. Reverse the direction by forcibly extending the left hip and knee, bringing the leg backward until you return to the start position. Perform the exercise with your right leg and then alternate legs until you reach the desired number of reps.

Brad's Training Tips

- Make sure your knee travels in line with the plane of your toes.
- Focus on dropping down on your rear leg—this keeps the front knee from pushing too far forward, which can place undue stress on the joint capsule.

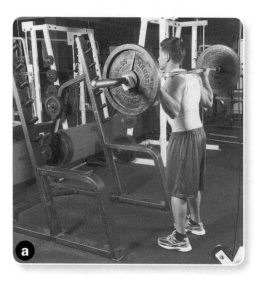
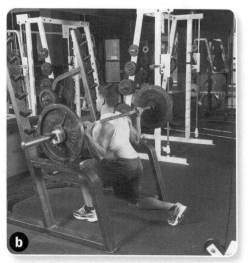

Dumbbell Lunge

Target

This move targets the quads and glutes. Secondary emphasis is on the hamstrings.

Start

Grasp two dumbbells and allow them to hang down by your sides, palms facing your body. Assume a shoulder-width stance and hold your shoulders back and your chin up.

Movement

Keeping your core tight, take a long step forward with your right leg, slowly lowering your body by flexing your right knee and hip in the process. Continue your descent until your left knee is almost in contact with the floor. Reverse the direction by forcibly extending the right hip and knee, bringing the leg backward until you return to the start position. Perform the exercise with your left leg and then alternate legs until you reach the desired number of reps.

Brad's Training Tips

- Make sure your front knee travels in line with the plane of your toes.
- Focus on dropping down on your rear leg—this keeps the front knee from pushing too far forward, which can place undue stress on the joint capsule.
- Look up as you perform the move—this helps prevent rounding at the upper spine.

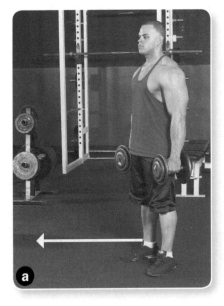
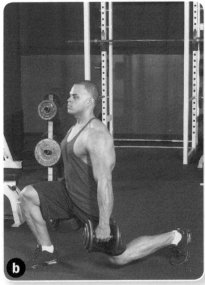

Dumbbell Reverse Lunge

Target

This move targets the quads and glutes. Secondary emphasis is on the hamstrings.

Start

Grasp two dumbbells and allow them to hang down by your sides, palms facing your body. Assume a shoulder-width stance and hold your shoulders back and your chin up.

Movement

Keeping your core tight, take a long step backward with your left leg, slowly lowering your body by flexing your right knee and hip in the process. Continue your descent until your left knee is almost in contact with the floor. Reverse the direction by forcibly extending the right hip and knee, bringing your right leg forward until you return to the start position. Repeat the exercise with your right leg and then alternate legs until you reach the desired number of reps.

Brad's Training Tips

- A longer stride emphasizes more of the glutes; a shorter stride targets the quads.
- Look up as you perform the move—this helps prevent rounding at the upper spine.

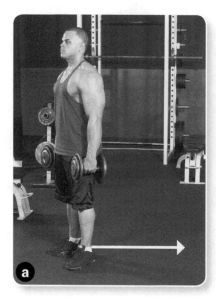
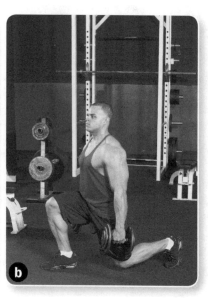

Dumbbell Side Lunge

Target

This move targets the muscles of the lower body, particularly the adductors of the inner thigh.

Start

Assume a wide stance, approximately one foot (0.3 m) or more past the width of your shoulders. Grasp two dumbbells and hold them at your sides.

Movement

Keeping your left leg straight, slowly bend your right knee out to the side until your right thigh is parallel with the floor. Forcefully rise back up and immediately repeat the exercise to your left. Alternate legs until you reach the desired number of reps.

Brad's Training Tips

- Make sure your front knee travels in line with the plane of your toes.
- Focus on dropping down on your rear leg—this keeps the front knee from pushing too far forward, which can place undue stress on the joint capsule.
- Look up as you perform the move—this helps prevent rounding at the upper spine.

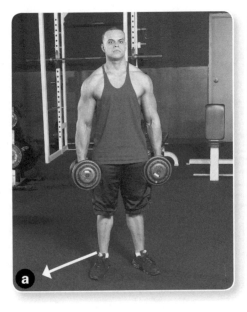 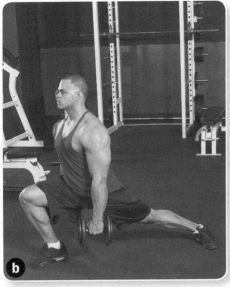

Dumbbell Step-Up

Target

This move targets the quads and glutes. Secondary emphasis is on the hamstrings.

Start

Grasp a pair of dumbbells and allow them to hang at your sides. Stand with your feet approximately shoulder-width apart and face the side of a flat bench.

Movement

Pushing off your left leg, step up on the bench with your right foot and follow with your left foot so that both feet are flat on the bench. Step back down in the same order, first with your left foot and then with your right, and return to the start position. Alternate legs for the desired number of reps.

Brad's Training Tips

- A higher step increases stimulation of the glutes.
- Look up as you perform the move—this helps prevent rounding at the upper spine.

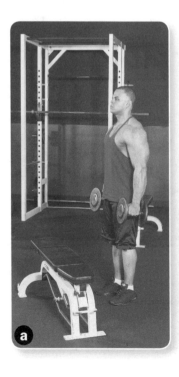
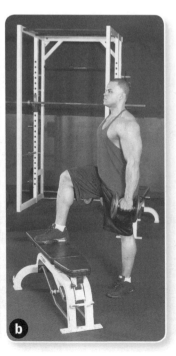
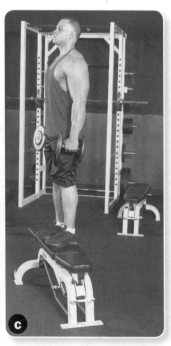

Barbell Front Squat

Target

This move targets the quads and glutes. Secondary emphasis is on the hamstrings. Particular emphasis is on the muscles of the frontal thighs.

Start

Rest a straight bar across your upper chest, holding it in place with both hands. Assume a shoulder-width stance and turn your feet slightly outward. Hold your shoulders back and your chin up.

Movement

Keeping your core tight, slowly lower your body until your thighs are parallel with the floor. Your lower back should be slightly arched and your heels should stay in contact with the floor at all times. When you reach a "seated" position, reverse the direction by straightening your legs and return to the start position.

Brad's Training Tips

- Your knees should travel in the same plane as your toes at all times.
- Your heels should stay in contact with the floor at all times. If you have trouble keeping your heels down, place a 1-inch (2.5 cm) block of wood or a weight plate under them.
- Wrap a towel around the bar if it feels uncomfortable on your chest.

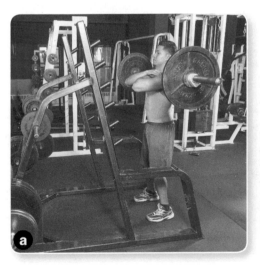
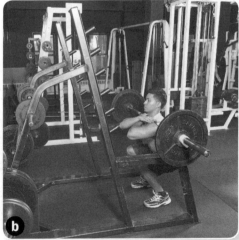

Barbell Back Squat

Target

This move targets the quads and glutes. Secondary emphasis is on the hamstrings.

Start

Rest a straight bar along the top of the shoulders at the base of your neck, grasping the bar with both hands. Assume a shoulder-width stance and slightly turn your feet outward.

Movement

Keeping your core tight, slowly lower your body until your thighs are parallel with the floor. Your lower back should be slightly arched and your heels should stay in contact with the floor at all times. When you reach a "seated" position, reverse the direction by straightening your legs and return to the start position.

Brad's Training Tips

- Your knees should travel in the same plane as your toes at all times.
- Your heels should stay in contact with the floor at all times. If you have trouble keeping your heels down, place a 1-inch (2.5 cm) block of wood or a weight plate under them.
- Wrap a towel around the bar if it feels uncomfortable on your neck.

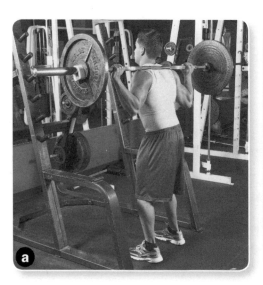
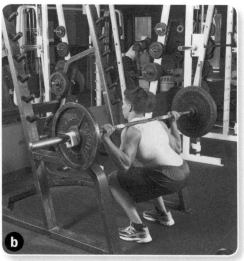

Barbell Split Squat

Target

This move targets the quads and glutes. Secondary emphasis is on the hamstrings.

Start

Rest a barbell across your shoulders, grasping the bar on both sides to maintain balance. Take a long stride forward with your left leg and raise your right heel so that your right foot is on its toes. Hold your shoulders back and your chin up.

Movement

Keeping your core tight, slowly lower your body by flexing your left knee and hip. Continue your descent until your right knee is almost in contact with the floor. Reverse the direction by forcibly extending your right hip and knee until you return to the start position. After you complete the desired number of reps, repeat the process with your right leg forward.

Brad's Training Tips

- Make sure your knee travels in line with the plane of your toes.
- Focus on dropping down on your rear leg—this keeps the front knee from pushing too far forward, which can place undue stress on the joint capsule.

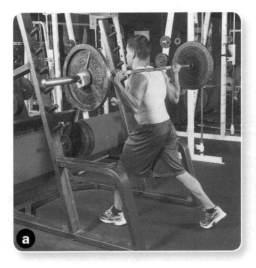
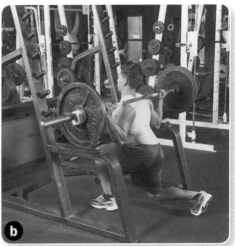

Bulgarian Squat

Target

This move targets the quads and glutes. Secondary emphasis is on the hamstrings.

Start

Grasp two dumbbells and allow your arms to hang down by your sides, palms facing your hips. Stand approximately 2 feet (0.6 m) in front of a raised object (such as a bench or chair) and place your left instep on top of the object. Your back should be straight. Hold your head up and your chest out.

Movement

Keeping your front foot flat on the floor, slowly lower your body until your right thigh is approximately parallel with the floor. Your lower back should be slightly arched and your right heel should stay in contact with the floor at all times. When you reach a "seated" position, reverse the direction by straightening your right leg and return to the start position. After you complete the desired number of reps, repeat the process on the opposite side.

Brad's Training Tips

■ You can increase the difficulty of the exercise by raising the height of the bench.

■ Look up as you perform the move—this helps prevent rounding at the upper spine.

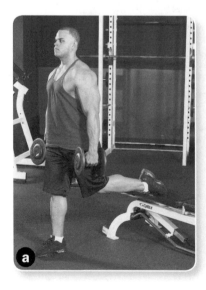 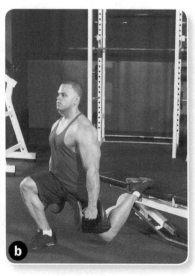

Leg Press

Target

This move targets the glutes and the quads. Secondary emphasis is on the hamstrings.

Start

Sit back in the seat of an angled leg press machine. Place your feet on the footplate and assume a shoulder-width stance. Keeping your toes angled slightly outward, straighten your legs and unlock the carriage-release bars located on the sides of the machine.

Movement

Keeping your back pressed firmly against the padded seat, slowly lower your legs and bring your knees in toward your chest. Without bouncing at the bottom of the movement, press the weight up in a controlled fashion and contract your quads. Stop just before you lock your knees.

Brad's Training Tip

- Placing your feet high on the footplate increases stimulation of the glutes; placing your feet low emphasizes the quads.

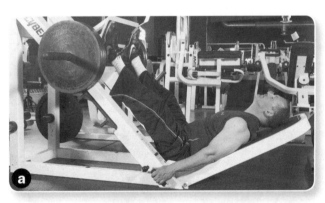

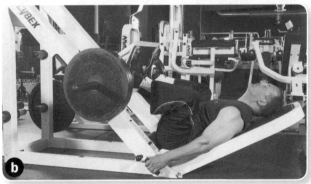

Deadlift

Target

This moves targets the entire lower-body musculature. It also works a number of upper-body muscles.

Start

Assume a shoulder-width stance a few inches (12 to 15 cm) in front of a barbell that rests on the floor. Bend your knees and, placing your hands just outside of your legs, grasp the bar with an alternating grip (one hand over the bar, the other hand under the bar). Keep your spine neutral.

Movement

Keeping your head up, chest out, and straight arms, drive the weight up by forcefully extending your legs and hips. Contract your glutes as you reach the top of the lift and then return to the start position.

Brad's Training Tips

- Keep your shins as close to the bar as possible when you lift—this maximizes leverage by shortening the distance of gravity.
- Do not hyperextend your lower back at the top of the lift. Rather, your body should form a straight line as you contract your glutes.
- You can use lifting straps if you have trouble holding the weight.

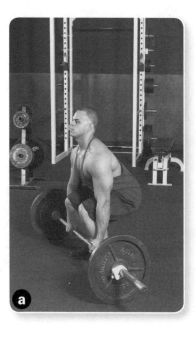 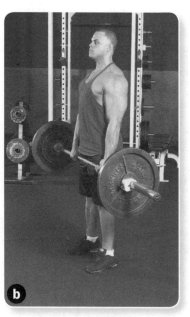

Good Morning

Target

This move targets the glutes and hamstrings.

Start

Rest a barbell across your shoulders, grasping the bar on both sides to maintain balance. Assume a shoulder-width stance. Hold your head up and keep your knees and back straight.

Movement

Keeping your lower back taut throughout the movement, slowly bend forward at the hips until your body is roughly parallel with the floor. In a controlled fashion, reverse the direction and contract your glutes as you rise up along the same path back to the start position.

Brad's Training Tips

- Wrap a towel around the bar if it feels uncomfortable on your neck.
- Move only at the hips, not the waist. Any spinal movement places the vertebrae at risk of injury. The long moment arm (the distance between the resistance and the axis of rotation) in this exercise makes a tight core critical.
- This move is not recommended for those with an existing lower-back injury.

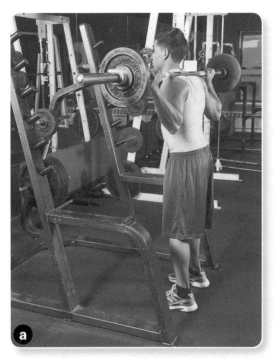
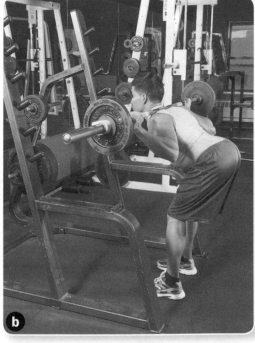

Sissy Squat

Target

This move targets the quads, particularly the rectus femoris.

Start

Assume a shoulder-width stance. Grasp a stationary object with one hand and rise up onto your toes.

Movement

In one motion, slowly slant your torso back, bend your knees, and lower your body. Thrust your knees forward as you descend and lean back until your torso is as close to parallel with the floor as possible. Then, reverse the direction and rise up until you reach the start position.

Brad's Training Tips

- Make sure you remain on your toes throughout the move—keeping your feet planted can result in injury to the knees.
- If the exercise becomes too easy and you are not challenged within your given rep range, you can hold a dumbbell or weight plate to your chest for added intensity.
- This move is contraindicated for those with existing knee injury.

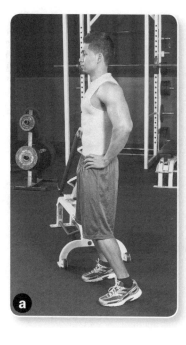
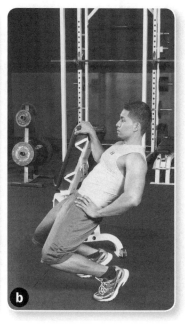

Barbell Stiff-Legged Deadlift

Target

This move targets the glutes and hamstrings.

Start

Stand with your feet about shoulder-width apart with knees straight and core tight. Grasp a straight bar and let it hang in front of your body.

Movement

Keeping your knees straight and core tight, slowly bend forward at the hips and lower the barbell until you feel an intense stretch in your hamstrings. Then, reverse the direction and contract your glutes as you rise up to the start position.

Brad's Training Tips

- Bend forward only at the hips, not the lower back. The action is purely hip extension, and any spinal movement places the vertebrae at risk of injury.
- Standing on a box, which many people do, is necessary only if you can touch your toes without flexing your spine—a feat very few people are capable of.

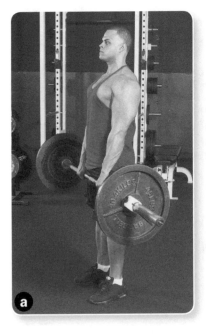
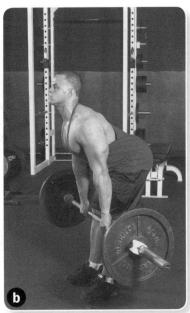

Dumbbell Stiff-Legged Deadlift

Target

This move targets the glutes and hamstrings.

Start

Stand with your feet about shoulder-width apart with knees straight and core tight. Grasp a pair of dumbbells and let them hang in front of your body.

Movement

Keeping your knees straight and core tight, slowly bend forward at the hips and lower the dumbbells until you feel an intense stretch in your hamstrings. Then, reverse the direction and forcefully contract your glutes as you rise up to the start position.

Brad's Training Tips

- Bend forward only at the hips, not the lower back. The action is purely hip extension, and any spinal movement places the vertebrae at risk of injury.
- Standing on a box, which many people do, is necessary only if you can touch your toes without flexing your spine—a feat very few people are capable of.

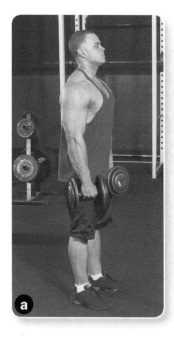
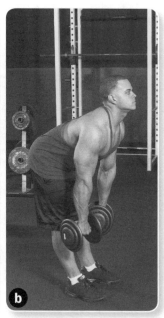

Cable Glute Kickback

Target

This move targets the glutes, particularly the gluteus maximus and hamstrings.

Start

Attach a cuff to a low-pulley apparatus and secure the cuff to your right ankle. Face the machine and grasp a sturdy object for support.

Movement

Keeping your upper body motionless and your right leg straight, bring your right foot back as far as comfortably possible. Contract your glutes and slowly return to the start position. After you complete the desired number of reps on your right side, repeat with your left leg.

Brad's Training Tip

- To decrease activation of the hamstrings and thereby increase activation of the glutes, bend the working knee slightly while performing the move.

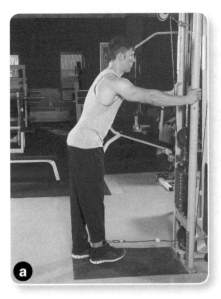
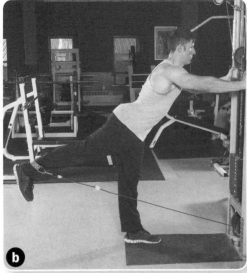

Hyperextension

Target

This move targets the glutes and hamstrings.

Start

Lie prone on a Roman chair. Hook your feet securely under the roller pads and rest your pelvis on the bench pad. Cross your arms over your chest.

Movement

Keeping your lower body stable and your head up, lift your chest and shoulders up until your body is parallel with the floor. Contract your glutes and return along the same path to the start position.

Brad's Training Tips

- Don't move your head during the movement—doing so can cause injury to your neck.
- Don't hyperextend your lower back—this can cause lumbar injury.
- To increase the level of difficulty, hold a weight plate against your chest as you perform the move.

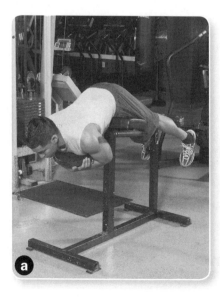

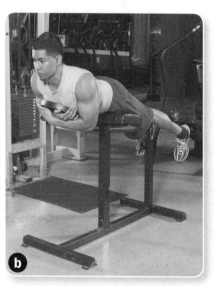

Reverse Hyperextension

Target

This move targets the glutes and hamstrings.

Start

Lie prone on a Roman chair and grasp the metal post under the roller pads. Rest your chest and abdomen on the bench pad. Your legs should hang down as far as possible without touching the floor.

Movement

Keeping your arms fixed, lift your legs up until your ankles and the back of your head are in a straight line. Contract your glutes and return along the same path back to the start position.

Brad's Training Tips

- Your knees should remain straight throughout the move. Don't use momentum by flexing and then whipping the lower legs straight.
- Don't hyperextend the back—this can cause lumbar injury.
- If the move becomes easy, attach leg weights to your ankles.

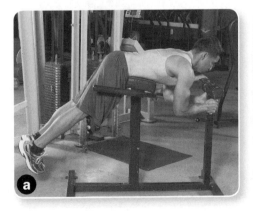
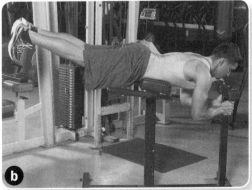

Leg Extension

Target

This move targets the quads.

Start

Sit upright in a leg extension machine so that the underside of your knees touches the edge of the seat. Bend your knees and place your instep under the roller pad located at the bottom of the machine. Grasp the machine's handles for support, tighten your core, and straighten your back.

Movement

Keeping your thighs and upper body immobile, lift your feet up until your legs are almost parallel with the floor. Contract your quads and then reverse the direction and return to the start position.

Brad's Training Tips

- Because of the extreme shear forces associated with this move, it is not recommended for those with knee problems. When in doubt, check with your physician.
- Turning your feet in or out offers no benefit. Keep them pointed straight ahead.

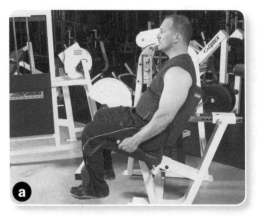 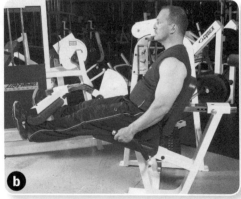

One-Leg Extension

Target

This move targets the quads.

Start

Sit upright in a leg extension machine so that the underside of your knees touches the edge of the seat. Bend your right knee and place your right instep under the roller pad located at the bottom of the machine. Keep your left leg back so that it is off the roller pad. Grasp the machine's handles for support, tighten your core, and straighten your back.

Movement

Keeping your thighs and upper body immobile, lift your right foot up until your right lower leg is almost parallel with the floor. Contract your quads and then reverse the direction and return to the start position. After you complete the desired number of reps, repeat the process on your left side.

Brad's Training Tips

- Because of the extreme shear forces associated with this move, it is not recommended for those with knee problems. When in doubt, check with your physician.
- Turning your feet in or out offers no benefit. Keep them pointed straight ahead.

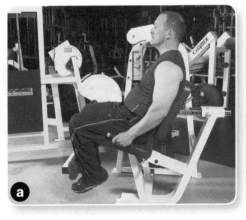
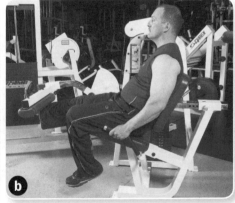

Lying Leg Curl

Target

This move targets the hamstrings.

Start

Lie facedown on a lying leg curl machine. Hook your heels under the roller pad. Grasp the handles (if available) or the bench pad for stability.

Movement

Keeping your thighs pressed against the bench surface, bend your knees and bring your feet up and toward your body, stopping just short of touching your feet to your butt or as close to that point as is comfortably possible. Contract your hamstrings and then reverse the direction and return to the start position.

Brad's Training Tip

■ Don't allow the moving weight stack to touch the nonmoving part of the weight stack at the start of the move—doing so takes tension off the hamstrings.

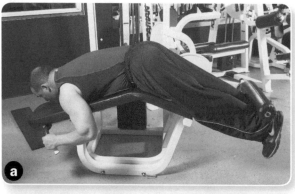

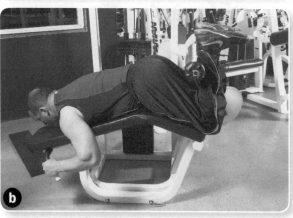

Machine Kneeling Leg Curl

Target

This move targets the hamstrings.

Start

Place your left knee on the knee pad of a kneeling leg curl machine and hook your right heel under the roller pad. Place your forearms on the restraint pads for support. Keep your back flat and your torso immobile throughout the move.

Movement

Bring your right foot up and toward your body, stopping just short of touching your foot to your butt or as close to that point as is comfortably possible. Contract your right hamstring and then reverse the direction and return to the start position. After you complete the desired number of reps, repeat the process on your left side.

Brad's Training Tip

■ Don't allow the moving weight stack to touch the nonmoving part of the weight stack at the start of the move—doing so takes tension off the hamstrings.

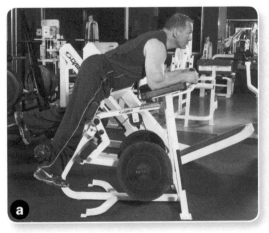
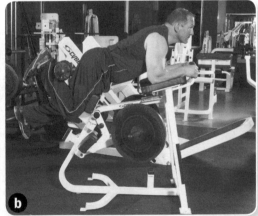

Machine Seated Leg Curl

Target

This move targets the hamstrings.

Start

Sit in a seated leg curl machine. Keep your back flat against the back rest and place your heels over the roller pads. Lower the leg restraint over your thighs.

Movement

Press your feet downward as far as comfortably possible. Contract your hamstrings when your knees are fully bent. Then, reverse the direction and return to the start position.

Brad's Training Tip

- Don't allow the moving weight stack to touch the nonmoving part of the weight stack at the start of the move—doing so takes tension off the hamstrings.

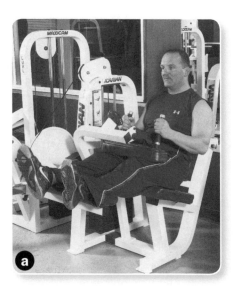
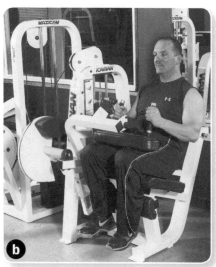

Toe Press

Target

This move targets the calf muscles.

Start

Sit upright in a leg-press machine and press your back firmly against the padded seat. Place the balls of your feet a comfortable distance apart on the bottom of the footplate, keeping your heels off the footplate. Straighten your legs, unlock the carriage-release bars, and drop your heels below your toes.

Movement

Keeping your knees immobile, press your toes as high up as you can until your ankles are fully extended. Contract your calves and then slowly reverse the direction and return to the start position.

Brad's Training Tips

- Never bounce during the stretched position of the move—this can cause severe injury to the Achilles tendon.
- Turning your toes outward can place increased emphasis on the middle head of the gastrocnemius; turning your toes inward can help target the lateral gastrocnemius head.

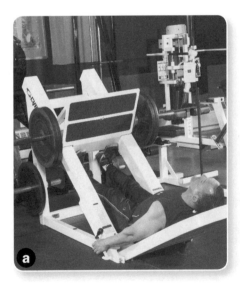
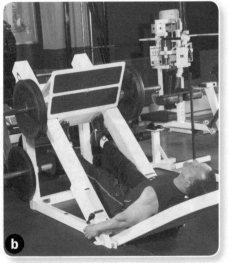

Machine Seated Calf Raise

Target

This move targets the calves, particularly the soleus muscle.

Start

Sit in a seated calf machine and place the restraint pads tightly across your thighs. Place the balls of your feet on the footplate and drop your heels as far below your toes as possible.

Movement

Rise as high as you can on your toes until your ankles are fully extended. Contract your calves and then slowly reverse the direction and return to the start position.

Brad's Training Tips

- Never bounce during the stretched position of the move—this can cause severe injury to the Achilles tendon.
- Because the gastrocnemius muscle is not very active in this exercise, it is best to keep your toes pointed straight ahead.

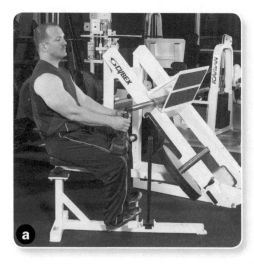
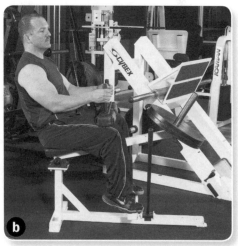

Machine Standing Calf Raise

Target

This move targets the calf muscles.

Start

Place your shoulders under the restraint pads of a standing calf machine. Place the balls of your feet on the footplate and drop your heels below your toes.

Movement

Rise as high as you can onto your toes until your ankles are fully extended. Contract your calves and then slowly reverse the direction and return to the start position.

Brad's Training Tips

- Never bounce during the stretched position of the move—this can cause severe injury to the Achilles tendon.
- Turning your toes outward can place increased emphasis on the middle head of the gastrocnemius; turning your toes inward can help to target the lateral head of the gastrocnemius.

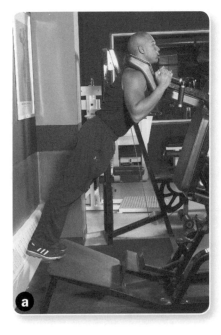
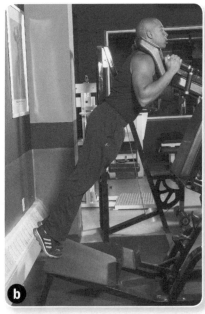

CHAPTER 6

MAX Break-In Routine

Make no mistake: The MAX Muscle Plan is a hard-core, muscle-building routine. As such, it's intended for those who have at least some lifting experience, ideally six months or more. If you lack the requisite experience, the program is likely to overwhelm your recuperative abilities and rapidly lead to an overtrained state.

If you're relatively new to resistance training or perhaps coming back from a prolonged layoff from lifting, don't worry. I created the MAX break-in routine with you in mind. It's a conditioning routine that is designed to prepare your body to deal with the rigorous nature of MAX training.

If you're a seasoned, active lifter, feel free to skip this chapter and proceed with the MAX strength phase of the program. Before doing so, however, be sure to honestly assess your ability to handle intensive exercise. Should you attempt MAX training before you're ready, you're bound to become overtrained. This will set your progress back, potentially for weeks if not months. If you have any doubt about whether you're prepared for the program, err on the side of caution and start with the break-in routine. Better safe than sorry.

PROGRAM PROTOCOL

The MAX break-in routine is a total-body workout in which you train all the major muscles during each session. It is an eight-week mesocycle and consists of two training blocks. Each block includes four one-week microcycles.

Block 1 is an initial break-in routine. It's for those who have no experience whatsoever or who are coming back after a long layoff from lifting. During this block, multijoint movements are incorporated whenever possible, with the exception of exercises for the arms and calves. Exercise selection is very limited, and you'll perform the same basic movements during each session. This might seem rudimentary and a tad boring; however, it is an important conditioning strategy. The primary adaptations during the early stages of training involve your nervous system; muscle hypertrophy is almost nonexistent for the first couple of months. During the early stages of training, your body gets used to new movement patterns and finds the most economical way to perform a given exercise. Focusing on a limited number of movements facilitates skill acquisition and allows coordinated motor programs to develop.

You'll train exclusively with high repetitions (15-20 per set) during this block. The higher rep range affords more practice and helps ingrain movement patterns into your subconscious mind. Moreover, it takes the onus away from generating high amounts of force and allows you to concentrate on proper technique. Remember, your sole objective is to get a feel for exercise performance. Once you learn the basic movements, muscle development will follow.

Block 2 is an extended break-in that builds on the skills you acquired during the initial break-in routine. At this point you'll have developed basic neuromuscular coordination and solidified technique in fundamental movement patterns. During block 2 you'll expand your ability to perform these movement patterns with a greater variety of exercises with varying levels of intensity. To accomplish this task, you'll follow a fairly traditional undulating periodization schedule that rotates between light, medium, and heavy weeks. You'll use a combination of single- and multijoint movements that change from one workout to the next. Sets will require increasingly greater levels of effort, and the final set takes you to the point of momentary muscle failure.

Throughout the break-in phase, perform repetitions in a deliberate, controlled fashion. Aim for a cadence of about one to two seconds on the concentric portion of each rep and approximately two to three seconds on the eccentric portion. Never speed up tempo at the expense of proper form. This will only cause you to develop bad habits that can be difficult to rectify in the future.

PROGRAM SPECIFICS

As noted, the MAX strength phase comprises two training blocks. Here are the particulars of each block.

Block 1

Block 1 is the initial break-in routine. It comprises four one-week microcycles. During the first three microcycles, you'll work out on three nonconsecutive days per week (e.g., Monday, Wednesday, and Friday) and train all the major muscle groups during each session. One exercise will be performed per muscle group. You'll perform three sets per exercise and take approximately one to two minutes of rest between sets. Intensity of all four microcycles should correspond to 15- to 20RM. Gradually increase effort on a weekly basis over the first three microcycles as follows.

During the first microcycle in block 1 (week 1 of the mesocycle), your level of effort on all sets should correspond to an RPE of 6, meaning that the lifts are somewhat hard. You should not struggle on any of the lifts. Rather, your goal is simply to get a feel for the movements and develop a sense of coordination between the working muscles. Rest intervals should be approximately one to two minutes between sets.

During the second microcycle of block 1 (week 2), your level of effort on all sets should correspond to an RPE of 7. The lifts should begin to get a little more difficult, but not to the extent that you struggle on the last couple reps. Concentrate on producing smooth, controlled movements to further develop neuromuscular coordination. Rest intervals should be approximately one to two minutes between sets.

During the third microcycle of block 1 (week 3), your level of effort on all sets should correspond to an RPE of 8 to 9, meaning that the lifts are very hard. At this level the weights should significantly tax your abilities. Do not train to all-out failure, however. Doing so will be counterproductive at this point. Keep your focus on hardwiring the neural circuitry between your brain and your muscles so that movements become second nature. Rest intervals should be approximately one to two minutes between sets.

The fourth microcycle in block 1 (week 4) constitutes an unloading phase. You'll train two days per week, allowing 72 hours between sessions (e.g., Monday and Thursday), and follow a total-body routine that works all the major muscle groups during each session. You'll perform one exercise of three sets per muscle group. Intensity will be 15 to 20RM. Sets should not be overly challenging. Aim for an RPE of 6 or so. If you struggle on the last few reps, lighten the weight! Rest intervals should be approximately one to two minutes between sets.

By the end of the fourth microcycle, you should be comfortable performing the exercises in good form. If so, progress to block 2. If not, repeat block 1 until you develop the necessary coordination and control for carrying out each movement.

Block 2

Block 2 is the extended break-in routine. Similar to block 1, it comprises four one-week microcycles. During the first three microcycles, you'll work out on three nonconsecutive days per week (e.g., Monday, Wednesday, and Friday) and train all the major muscle groups during each session. One exercise will be performed per muscle group. You'll perform three sets per exercise and take approximately one to two minutes of rest between sets. A variety of exercises are incorporated into the routine to facilitate greater acclimation to different movements. Intensity will increase each week over the course of the first three microcycles, and the last set of each exercise takes you to the point of muscle failure as follows.

The first microcycle in block 2 (week 5 of the mesocycle) targets an intensity corresponding to 15- to 20RM. Perform the first set at an RPE of about 7, perform the second set at an RPE of about 8 to 9, and take the final set to the point of concentric muscle failure. Rest intervals should be approximately 30 seconds between sets.

The second microcycle in block 2 (week 6) targets an intensity corresponding to 8- to 10RM (except the abs, which are trained with higher repetitions). Perform the first set at an RPE of about 7, perform the second set at an RPE of about 8 to 9, and take the final set to the point of concentric muscle failure. Rest intervals should be approximately one to two minutes between sets.

The third microcycle in block 2 (week 7) targets an intensity corresponding to 3- to 5RM (except the abs, which are trained with higher repetitions). Perform the first set at an RPE of about 7, perform the second set at an RPE of about 8 to 9, and take the final set to the point of concentric muscle failure. Rest intervals should be approximately three minutes between sets.

The fourth microcycle in block 2 (week 8) constitutes an unloading phase. You'll train two days per week, allowing 72 hours between session (e.g., Monday and Thursday), and follow a total-body routine that works all the major muscle groups during each session. You'll perform one exercise of three sets per muscle group. Intensity will be 15- to 20RM. Sets should not be overly challenging. Aim for an RPE of 6 or so. If you struggle on the last few reps, lighten the weight! Rest intervals should be approximately one to two minutes between sets.

I recommend that you repeat the extended break-in routine several times before initiating the MAX Muscle Plan. This helps ensure that you're fully prepared for the stresses of MAX training and diminishes the potential for becoming overtrained.

Table 6.1 summarizes the MAX break-in protocol, and sample routines (tables 6.2 through 6.9) are provided on the subsequent pages. These routines should serve as a basic template for constructing your workouts. Modify specific exercises according to your individual needs and abilities.

Table 6.1 Summary of MAX Break-In Routine

Training variable	Protocol
Repetitions	3-20
Sets	3 per exercise
Rest interval	30 sec to 3 min
Tempo	Concentric: 1-2 sec Eccentric: 2-3 sec
Frequency	3 days per week

Table 6.2 Break-In Week 1: Block 1 Microcycle 1

Perform these exercises at an RPE of 6.

Day	Target muscles	Exercises	Page #
Monday	Total body	Dumbbell chest press (3 sets @ 15-20RM)	45
		Dumbbell one-arm row (3 sets @ 15-20RM)	27
		Dumbbell shoulder press (3 sets @ 15-20RM)	76
		Dumbbell standing biceps curl (3 sets @ 15-20RM)	87
		Cable triceps press-down (3 sets @ 15-20RM)	107
		Barbell back squat (3 sets @ 15-20RM)	119
		Lying leg curl (3 sets @ 15-20RM)	133
		Machine standing calf raise (3 sets @ 15-20RM)	138
		Crunch (3 sets @ 15-20RM)	56
Tuesday	Off		
Wednesday	Total body	Dumbbell chest press (3 sets @ 15-20RM)	45
		Dumbbell one-arm row (3 sets @ 15-20RM)	27
		Dumbbell shoulder press (3 sets @ 15-20RM)	76
		Dumbbell standing biceps curl (3 sets @ 15-20RM)	87
		Cable triceps press-down (3 sets @ 15-20RM)	107
		Barbell back squat (3 sets @ 15-20RM)	119
		Lying leg curl (3 sets @ 15-20RM)	133
		Machine standing calf raise (3 sets @ 15-20RM)	138
		Crunch (3 sets @ 15-20RM)	56
Thursday	Off		
Friday	Total body	Dumbbell chest press (3 sets @ 15-20RM)	45
		Dumbbell one-arm row (3 sets @ 15-20RM)	27
		Dumbbell shoulder press (3 sets @ 15-20RM)	76
		Dumbbell standing biceps curl (3 sets @ 15-20RM)	87
		Cable triceps press-down (3 sets @ 15-20RM)	107
		Barbell back squat (3 sets @ 15-20RM)	119
		Lying leg curl (3 sets @ 15-20RM)	133
		Machine standing calf raise (3 sets @ 15-20RM)	138
		Crunch (3 sets @ 15-20RM)	56
Saturday	Off		
Sunday	Off		

Table 6.3 Break-In Week 2: Block 1 Microcycle 2

Perform these exercises at an RPE of 7.

Day	Target muscles	Exercises	Page #
Monday	Total body	Dumbbell chest press (3 sets @ 15-20RM)	45
		Dumbbell one-arm row (3 sets @ 15-20RM)	27
		Dumbbell shoulder press (3 sets @ 15-20RM)	76
		Dumbbell standing biceps curl (3 sets @ 15-20RM)	87
		Cable triceps press-down (3 sets @ 15-20RM)	107
		Barbell back squat (3 sets @ 15-20RM)	119
		Lying leg curl (3 sets @ 15-20RM)	133
		Machine standing calf raise (3 sets @ 15-20RM)	138
		Crunch (3 sets @ 15-20RM)	56
Tuesday	Off		
Wednesday	Total body	Dumbbell chest press (3 sets @ 15-20RM)	45
		Dumbbell one-arm row (3 sets @ 15-20RM)	27
		Dumbbell shoulder press (3 sets @ 15-20RM)	76
		Dumbbell standing biceps curl (3 sets @ 15-20RM)	87
		Cable triceps press-down (3 sets @ 15-20RM)	107
		Barbell back squat (3 sets @ 15-20RM)	119
		Lying leg curl (3 sets @ 15-20RM)	133
		Machine standing calf raise (3 sets @ 15-20RM)	138
		Crunch (3 sets @ 15-20RM)	56
Thursday	Off		
Friday	Total body	Dumbbell chest press (3 sets @ 15-20RM)	45
		Dumbbell one-arm row (3 sets @ 15-20RM)	27
		Dumbbell shoulder press (3 sets @ 15-20RM)	76
		Dumbbell standing biceps curl (3 sets @ 15-20RM)	87
		Cable triceps press-down (3 sets @ 15-20RM)	107
		Barbell back squat (3 sets @ 15-20RM)	119
		Lying leg curl (3 sets @ 15-20RM)	133
		Machine standing calf raise (3 sets @ 15-20RM)	138
		Crunch (3 sets @ 15-20RM)	56
Saturday	Off		
Sunday	Off		

Table 6.4 Break-In Week 3: Block 1 Microcycle 3

Perform these exercises at an RPE of 8 or 9.

Day	Target muscles	Exercises	Page #
Monday	Total body	Dumbbell chest press (3 sets @ 15-20RM)	45
		Dumbbell one-arm row (3 sets @ 15-20RM)	27
		Dumbbell shoulder press (3 sets @ 15-20RM)	76
		Dumbbell standing biceps curl (3 sets @ 15-20RM)	87
		Cable triceps press-down (3 sets @ 15-20RM)	107
		Barbell back squat (3 sets @ 15-20RM)	119
		Lying leg curl (3 sets @ 15-20RM)	133
		Machine standing calf raise (3 sets @ 15-20RM)	138
		Crunch (3 sets @ 15-20RM)	56
Tuesday	Off		
Wednesday	Total body	Dumbbell chest press (3 sets @ 15-20RM)	45
		Dumbbell one-arm row (3 sets @ 15-20RM)	27
		Dumbbell shoulder press (3 sets @ 15-20RM)	76
		Dumbbell standing biceps curl (3 sets @ 15-20RM)	87
		Cable triceps press-down (3 sets @ 15-20RM)	107
		Barbell back squat (3 sets @ 15-20RM)	119
		Lying leg curl (3 sets @ 15-20RM)	133
		Machine standing calf raise (3 sets @ 15-20RM)	138
		Crunch (3 sets @ 15-20RM)	56
Thursday	Off		
Friday	Total body	Dumbbell chest press (3 sets @ 15-20RM)	45
		Dumbbell one-arm row (3 sets @ 15-20RM)	27
		Dumbbell shoulder press (3 sets @ 15-20RM)	76
		Dumbbell standing biceps curl (3 sets @ 15-20RM)	87
		Cable triceps press-down (3 sets @ 15-20RM)	107
		Barbell back squat (3 sets @ 15-20RM)	119
		Lying leg curl (3 sets @ 15-20RM)	133
		Machine standing calf raise (3 sets @ 15-20RM)	138
		Crunch (3 sets @ 15-20RM)	56
Saturday	Off		
Sunday	Off		

Table 6.5 Break-In Week 4: Block 1 Microcycle 4

Perform these exercises at an RPE of 6.

Day	Target muscles	Exercises	Page #
Monday	Total body	Dumbbell chest press (3 sets @ 15-20RM)	45
		Dumbbell one-arm row (3 sets @ 15-20RM)	27
		Dumbbell shoulder press (3 sets @ 15-20RM)	76
		Dumbbell standing biceps curl (3 sets @ 15-20RM)	87
		Cable triceps press-down (3 sets @ 15-20RM)	107
		Barbell back squat (3 sets @ 15-20RM)	119
		Lying leg curl (3 sets @ 15-20RM)	133
		Machine standing calf raise (3 sets @ 15-20RM)	138
		Crunch (3 sets @ 15-20RM)	56
Tuesday	Off		
Wednesday	Off		
Thursday	Total body	Dumbbell chest press (3 sets @ 15-20RM)	45
		Dumbbell one-arm row (3 sets @ 15-20RM)	27
		Dumbbell shoulder press (3 sets @ 15-20RM)	76
		Dumbbell standing biceps curl (3 sets @ 15-20RM)	87
		Cable triceps press-down (3 sets @ 15-20RM)	107
		Barbell back squat (3 sets @ 15-20RM)	119
		Lying leg curl (3 sets @ 15-20RM)	133
		Machine standing calf raise (3 sets @ 15-20RM)	138
		Crunch (3 sets @ 15-20RM)	56
Friday	Off		
Saturday	Off		
Sunday	Off		

Table 6.6 Break-In Week 5: Block 2 Microcycle 1

Perform the first set of exercises at an RPE of about 7, perform the second set at an RPE of about 8 to 9, and take the final set to the point of concentric muscle failure. Rest 30 seconds between sets.

Day	Target muscles	Exercises	Page #
Monday	Total body	Barbell chest press (3 sets @ 15-20RM)	47
		Cable seated row (3 sets @ 15-20RM)	33
		Military press (3 sets @ 15-20RM)	75
		Barbell curl (3 sets @ 15-20RM)	95
		Nosebreaker (3 sets @ 15-20RM)	102
		Bulgarian squat (3 sets @ 15-20RM)	121
		Barbell stiff-legged deadlift (3 sets @ 15-20RM)	126
		Machine standing calf raise (3 sets @ 15-20RM)	138
		Cable rope kneeling crunch (3 sets @ 15-20RM)	61
Tuesday	Off		
Wednesday	Total body	Dumbbell incline press (3 sets @ 15-20RM)	43
		Lat pull-down (3 sets @ 15-20RM)	38
		Dumbbell lateral raise (3 sets @ 15-20RM)	78
		Dumbbell incline biceps curl (3 sets @ 15-20RM)	88
		Cable rope overhead triceps extension (3 sets @ 15-20RM)	101
		Barbell front squat (3 sets @ 15-20RM)	118
		Machine seated leg curl (3 sets @ 15-20RM)	135
		Machine seated calf raise (3 sets @ 15-20RM)	137
		Bicycle crunch (3 sets @ 15-20RM)	58
Thursday	Off		
Friday	Total body	Barbell incline press (3 sets @ 15-20RM)	46
		Barbell overhand bent row (3 sets @ 15-20RM)	30
		Cable upright row (3 sets @ 15-20RM)	86
		Cable curl (3 sets @ 15-20RM)	98
		Dumbbell overhead triceps extension (3 sets @ 15-20RM)	100
		Dumbbell lunge (3 sets @ 15-20RM)	114
		Good morning (3 sets @ 15-20RM)	124
		Toe press (3 sets @ 15-20RM)	136
		Reverse crunch (3 sets @ 15-20RM)	57
Saturday	Off		
Sunday	Off		

Table 6.7 Break-In Week 6: Block 2 Microcycle 2

Perform the first set of exercises at an RPE of about 7, perform the second set at an RPE of about 8 to 9, and take the final set to the point of concentric muscle failure. Rest 1 to 2 minutes between sets.

Day	Target muscles	Exercises	Page #
Monday	Total body	Barbell chest press (3 sets @ 8-10RM)	47
		Cable seated row (3 sets @ 8-10RM)	33
		Military press (3 sets @ 8-10RM)	75
		Barbell curl (3 sets @ 8-10RM)	95
		Nosebreaker (3 sets @ 8-10RM)	102
		Bulgarian squat (3 sets @ 8-10RM)	121
		Barbell stiff-legged deadlift (3 sets @ 8-10RM)	126
		Machine standing calf raise (3 sets @ 8-10RM)	138
		Cable rope kneeling crunch (3 sets @ 15-20RM)	61
Tuesday	Off		
Wednesday	Total body	Dumbbell incline press (3 sets @ 8-10RM)	43
		Lat pull-down (3 sets @ 8-10RM)	38
		Arnold press (3 sets @ 8-10RM)	74
		Dumbbell incline biceps curl (3 sets @ 8-10RM)	88
		Cable rope overhead triceps extension (3 sets @ 8-10RM)	101
		Barbell front squat (3 sets @ 8-10RM)	118
		Machine seated leg curl (3 sets @ 8-10RM)	135
		Machine seated calf raise (3 sets @ 8-10RM)	137
		Bicycle crunch (3 sets @ 15-20RM)	58
Thursday	Off		
Friday	Total body	Barbell incline press (3 sets @ 8-10RM)	46
		Barbell overhand bent row (3 sets @ 8-10RM)	30
		Cable upright row (3 sets @ 8-10RM)	86
		Cable curl (3 sets @ 8-10RM)	98
		Dumbbell overhead triceps extension (3 sets @ 8-10RM)	100
		Dumbbell lunge (3 sets @ 8-10RM)	114
		Good morning (3 sets @ 8-10RM)	124
		Toe press (3 sets @ 8-10RM)	136
		Reverse crunch (3 sets @ 15-20RM)	57
Saturday	Off		
Sunday	Off		

Table 6.8 Break-In Week 7: Block 2 Microcycle 3

Perform the first set at an RPE of about 7, perform the second set at an RPE of about 8 to 9, and take the final set to the point of concentric muscle failure. Rest approximately 3 minutes between sets.

Day	Target muscles	Exercises	Page #
Monday	Total body	Barbell chest press (3 sets @ 3-5RM)	47
		Cable seated row (3 sets @ 3-5RM)	33
		Military press (3 sets @ 3-5RM)	75
		Barbell curl (3 sets @ 3-5RM)	95
		Nosebreaker (3 sets @ 3-5RM)	102
		Bulgarian squat (3 sets @ 3-5RM)	121
		Barbell stiff-legged deadlift (3 sets @ 3-5RM)	126
		Machine standing calf raise (3 sets @ 3-5RM)	138
		Cable rope kneeling crunch (3 sets @ 15-20RM)	61
Tuesday	Off		
Wednesday	Total body	Dumbbell incline press (3 sets @ 3-5RM)	43
		Lat pull-down (3 sets @ 3-5RM)	38
		Arnold press (3 sets @ 3-5RM)	74
		Dumbbell incline biceps curl (3 sets @ 3-5RM)	88
		Cable rope overhead triceps extension (3 sets @ 3-5RM)	101
		Barbell front squat (3 sets @ 3-5RM)	118
		Machine seated leg curl (3 sets @ 3-5RM)	135
		Machine seated calf raise (3 sets @ 3-5RM)	137
		Bicycle crunch (3 sets @ 15-20RM)	58
Thursday	Off		
Friday	Total body	Barbell incline press (3 sets @ 3-5RM)	46
		Barbell overhand bent row (3 sets @ 3-5RM)	30
		Cable upright row (3 sets @ 3-5RM)	86
		Cable curl (3 sets @ 3-5RM)	98
		Dumbbell overhead triceps extension (3 sets @ 3-5RM)	100
		Dumbbell lunge (3 sets @ 3-5RM)	114
		Good morning (3 sets @ 3-5RM)	124
		Toe press (3 sets @ 3-5RM)	136
		Reverse crunch (3 sets @ 15-20RM)	57
Saturday	Off		
Sunday	Off		

Table 6.9 Break-In Week 8: Block 2 Microcycle 4

Perform these exercises at RPE of 6.

Day	Target muscles	Exercises	Page #
Monday	Total body	Dumbbell chest press (3 sets @ 15-20RM)	45
		Dumbbell one-arm row (3 sets @ 15-20RM)	27
		Dumbbell shoulder press (3 sets @ 15-20RM)	76
		Dumbbell standing biceps curl (3 sets @ 15-20RM)	87
		Cable triceps press-down (3 sets @ 15-20RM)	107
		Barbell back squat (3 sets @ 15-20RM)	119
		Lying leg curl (3 sets @ 15-20RM)	133
		Machine standing calf raise (3 sets @ 15-20RM)	138
		Crunch (3 sets @ 15-20RM)	56
Tuesday	Off		
Wednesday	Off		
Thursday	Total body	Barbell incline press (3 sets @ 15-20RM)	46
		Barbell overhand bent row (3 sets @ 15-20RM)	30
		Military press (3 sets @ 15-20RM)	75
		Cable curl (3 sets @ 15-20RM)	98
		Nosebreaker (3 sets @ 15-20RM)	102
		Barbell front squat (3 sets @ 15-20RM)	118
		Barbell stiff-legged deadlift (3 sets @ 15-20RM)	126
		Machine seated calf raise (3 sets @ 15-20RM)	137
		Cable rope kneeling crunch (3 sets @ 15-20RM)	61
Friday	Off		
Saturday	Off		
Sunday	Off		

CHAPTER 7

MAX Strength Phase

The MAX Muscle Plan begins with a MAX strength phase. During this phase you'll focus on lifting heavy weights in a low repetition range. The goal here is to get as strong as possible; increasing muscle size is of secondary concern at this point.

Why is it important to build strength when the overall goal is to maximize muscle development? The short answer is that getting stronger ultimately fosters better muscle growth. Quite simply, if you aren't physically strong, muscle development is bound to suffer.

I equate the process to building a house. Before erecting the frame of the house and laying down the hardwood flooring you must first construct a rock-solid foundation. Without a strong foundation, the house will ultimately crumble. Similarly, to achieve maximal muscle development you must build your body on a foundation of strength. Stronger muscles allow you to use heavier weights—and thus generate greater muscle tension—in the moderate repetition ranges that optimally stimulate hypertrophy. By increasing muscle tension without compromising metabolic stress, you set the stage for enhanced growth.

The most important adaptation to heavy lifting is an improvement in the response of your nervous system. You see, muscles are innervated—that is, activated—by nerve cells called neurons, which transmit electrical and chemical signals to a given number of fibers within a muscle. A single neuron and all the corresponding fibers it innervates are called a motor unit. The major muscles in your body are innervated by multiple motor units, often many thousands.

How does all this physiology relate to muscle growth? The ability of your muscles to exert force is governed by three distinct neural mechanisms: recruitment, rate coding, and synchronization. Let's take a brief look at how heavy strength training affects each of these factors.

Recruitment refers to the ability of your nervous system to activate motor units. Recruitment is generally governed by the size principle, which suggests that smaller motor units (primarily made up of endurance-oriented slow-twitch fibers) are recruited first and that larger motor units (primarily made up of strength-oriented fast-twitch fibers) are progressively recruited thereafter if and when additional force is required. Although many studies show that advanced trainees are able to recruit all available fibers at approximately 80 percent of 1RM, some believe that heavy weight training may help condition stubborn high-threshold motor units, thereby allowing their recruitment at lower percentages of 1RM. This leads to greater muscle fatigue across the full spectrum of fibers and thus greater muscle growth.

Rate coding refers to the frequency at which nerve impulses are stimulated during a lift. Nerve impulses that fire with a high frequency produce more muscle tension than do lower frequency impulses. Rate coding is widely considered the most important determinant of your ability to produce force. The good news is that heavy strength training increases the rate at which nerve impulses fire, and it can extend the firing period. The upshot is a greater sustained muscle tension during your lifts.

Synchronization refers to the coordinated timing between different motor units within a muscle (intramuscular coordination) or between different synergists (intermuscular coordination). As an analogy, think of synchronization as similar to a symphony orchestra. If the string section is not in sync with the percussion section or the violins are not in sync with each other, the end result is a hodgepodge of sounds. To produce sweet music, all the instruments must play harmoniously. Similarly, if the impulses reaching different motor units are out of phase, then muscle force is compromised. Fibers must contract as a unit in precise accord to maximize force production. Heavy lifting helps foster both intramuscular and intermuscular harmony in the fibers within both the target muscles and the stabilizing muscles.

By enhancing the efficiency of recruitment, rate coding, and synchronization, the MAX strength phase lays the groundwork for future muscle growth. It provides a strong base on which to build your body. As long as you follow the program in a step-by-step fashion, you will maximize muscle development during the MAX muscle phase.

PROGRAM PROTOCOL

The MAX strength phase is an eight week, high-intensity mesocycle that consists of two training blocks. Each block includes four one-week microcycles. Block 1 uses a total-body routine that works all the major muscles during each session, and block 2 uses an upper–lower split routine. Blocks are structured to progressively increase training volume over the course of the mesocycle while maintaining intensity levels.

With a few exceptions, you'll train in a range of one to five reps and take three to five minutes of rest between sets. Three sets are performed per exercise. The goal is to optimize force production by lifting heavy and hard. Realize, though, that constantly grinding out reps at near-maximal intensities really takes a toll on the body by overtaxing your neuromuscular system and overstressing your joints. To counteract these potential negative effects, intensity and volume are carefully manipulated throughout the training cycle and periods of unloading are interspersed at regimented points to allow adequate recuperation. What's more, training to failure is limited to just a few select sets; if you perform more than a few, you risk overtraining.

Lifts can be categorized as either primary exercises or accessory exercises. Primary exercises are multijoint movements that tax the prime movers and require a significant contribution from the muscles that work with the prime movers (synergists) and the muscles that stabilize the body during the performance of the exercise (stabilizers). In other words, they involve large amounts of total-body muscle mass. Examples include variations of squats, rows, and presses. These movements lend themselves to maximal or near-maximal lifts and thus are most conducive to optimizing increases in absolute strength.

Accessory exercises, on the other hand, are generally single-joint movements that involve working smaller amounts of muscle mass. In the context of the MAX strength phase, accessory exercises help rectify muscle imbalances by preventing weak links from forming in the kinetic chain. By their nature, primary exercises tend to stress some muscles more than others. In the squat, for example, hamstring activity is only about 50 percent that of the quadriceps. If you do not perform direct hamstring work, chances are you will become quad dominant and have impaired muscle symmetry. Thus, consider accessory exercises to be complementary movements that fill in the muscular gaps left by primary exercises. One caveat: Because accessory exercises place greater stress on joints, they tend to be incompatible with the use of very heavy loads. Hence, target a moderate repetition range of six to eight reps per set for these movements.

Exercise selection is more limited in the MAX strength phase than in the other phases of the program. Although exercise variety is important for maximizing muscle hypertrophy, it is less important with respect to strength development. The reason? Consistently training the same lifts hardwires neuromuscular patterns, thus enhancing both intra- and inter-muscular coordination. Because strength gains highly depend on neuromuscular efficiency, strength is best maximized by performing the same basic movements on a regular basis.

You should regulate tempo on both the concentric and eccentric portions of each rep. Concentrically, your objective is to lift as explosively as possible. Given that intensity is close to maximum (the target repetition range of one to five reps), this is easier said than done. You can exert all your effort into producing force, but the weights won't move very fast. This isn't of concern. As long as your intent is to lift explosively, you'll derive strength-related benefits. On the other hand, perform eccentric repetitions more slowly. Aim for a cadence of approximately two to three seconds. The most important consideration is to stay under control so that you do not compromise form. Never bounce at the bottom of a movement; you might eke out an extra rep or two, but you'll overstress your joints in a way that is bound to lead to injury.

You'll notice that the arms and abs are not trained directly in the MAX strength phase. Before you cry heresy, hear out my rationale. Remember that the goal of this phase is to get strong. Because you have a limited amount of training time, you need to center all of your energies on the large muscle group lifts that contribute most to increases in strength. The arms and abs don't fall into this category, and training them directly would only take away valuable energy that you should reserve for maximal strength development.

In case you're worried that these muscles will somehow shrivel up if you don't work them directly, rest easy. The biceps and triceps are heavily involved in all of the structural lifts and many of the assistance lifts, and the muscles of the core act as stabilizers in virtually every exercise you perform. Hence, they receive ample work throughout the MAX strength mesocycle—more than enough to maintain or even improve development. And rest assured that you will blitz these muscle groups during the later phases of the program to achieve the coveted peaked biceps and six-pack of abs.

PROGRAM SPECIFICS

As noted, the MAX strength phase is an eight-week mesocycle made up of two training blocks. Each block uses a technique called step loading in which intensity progressively increases over each of the first three weeks. The fourth week consists of an unloading microcycle of low-intensity, low-volume training. The unloading periods restore and rejuvenate muscles and joints and ultimately potentiate muscular supercompensation. Here are the particulars of each block.

Block 1

Block 1 is made up of four one-week microcycles. During the first three microcycles, you'll work out on three nonconsecutive days per week (e.g., Monday, Wednesday, and Friday) and follow a total-body routine that trains all the major muscle groups during every session. One exercise will be performed per muscle group. You'll perform three sets per exercise and take approximately three to five minutes between sets. Intensity is carried out using the following step-loading progression.

The first microcycle in block 1 (week 1 of the mesocycle) targets an intensity corresponding to 4- to 5RM. Your level of effort on all sets should correspond to an RPE of 8, meaning that the lifts are very taxing but do not progress to all-out muscle failure.

The second microcycle in block 1 (week 2) targets an intensity corresponding to 2- to 3RM. Your level of effort on all sets should correspond to an RPE of 9, meaning that the lifts are extremely taxing but do not progress to all-out muscle failure.

The third microcycle in block 1 (week 3) targets an intensity corresponding to 1- to 5RM in a descending-set fashion. The first set targets a 4- to 5RM, the second set targets a 2- to 3RM, and the final set targets a maximal lift at 1RM. Perform the first set (i.e., 4-5RM) at an RPE of 8, perform the second set (i.e., 2-3RM) at an RPE of 9, and take the final maximal set (i.e., 1RM) to the point of concentric muscle failure.

The fourth microcycle in block 1 (week 4) is an unloading phase. You'll train two days per week, allowing 72 hours between sessions (e.g., Monday and Thursday), and follow a total-body routine that works all the major muscle groups during each session. You'll perform one exercise of three sets per muscle group. Intensity will be 15- to 20RM. Sets should not be overly challenging. Aim for an RPE of 7 or so. If you struggle on the last few reps, lighten the weight!

Block 2

Block 2 is made up of four one-week microcycles. During the first three microcycles, you'll train four days per week using a sequence of either two on, one off, two on, two off (e.g., Monday, Tuesday, Thursday, and Friday) or two on, one off, one on, one off, one on, one off (e.g., Monday, Tuesday, Thursday, and Saturday). Training incorporates a two-day split that works the upper body on day 1 and the lower body on day 2. The number of exercises per muscle group increases to include both a structural exercise and a corresponding assistance exercise. You'll perform three sets per exercise and take approximately three to five minutes between sets on the structural exercises and two minutes of rest on the assistance exercises. Intensity is carried out using the same step-loading progression as in block 1. Thus, volume increases while intensity remains constant.

The first microcycle in block 2 (week 5 of the mesocycle) targets an intensity corresponding to 4- to 5RM for the structural exercises and 6- to 8RM for the assistance exercises. Your level of effort on all sets should correspond to an RPE of 7 to 8, meaning that the lifts are taxing but not overly stressful.

The second microcycle in block 2 (week 6) targets an intensity corresponding to 2- to 3RM for the structural exercises and 6- to 8RM for the assistance exercises. Your level of effort on all sets should correspond to an RPE of 8 to 9, meaning that the lifts are very taxing but do not progress to the point of complete muscle failure.

The third microcycle in block 2 (week 7) targets an intensity corresponding to 1- to 5RM in a descending-set fashion for the structural exercises. Thus, the first set for each structural exercise targets a 4- to 5RM, the second set targets a 2- to 3RM, and the final set targets a maximal lift at 1RM. On these sets, perform the first set (i.e., 4-5RM) at an RPE of 8, perform the second set (i.e., 2-3RM) at an RPE of 9, and take the final maximal set (i.e., 1RM) to the point of concentric muscle failure. Assistance exercises will maintain a 6- to 8RM for all sets, and effort should correspond to an RPE of approximately 8 to 9. Do not go to failure on the assistance exercises.

The fourth microcycle in block 2 (week 8) is an unloading phase. You'll train two days per week, allowing 72 hours between sessions (e.g., Monday and Thursday), and follow a total-body routine that works all the major muscle groups during each session. You'll perform one exercise of three sets per muscle group. Intensity will be 15- to 20RM. Sets should not be overly challenging. Aim for an RPE of 7 or so. If you struggle on the last few reps, lighten the weight!

Table 7.1 summarizes the MAX strength phase protocol, and sample routines (tables 7.2 through 7.9) are provided on the subsequent pages. These routines should serve as a basic template for constructing your workouts. Modify specific exercises according to your individual needs and abilities.

Table 7.1 Summary of MAX Strength Protocol

Training variable	Protocol
Repetitions	Structural exercises: 1-5
	Assistance exercises: 6-8
Sets	3 per exercise
Rest interval	Structural exercises: 3-5 min
	Assistance exercises: 2 min
Tempo	Concentric: explosive
	Eccentric: 2-3 sec
Frequency	3-4 days per week

Table 7.2 Strength Phase Week 1: Block 1 Microcycle 1

Perform these exercises at an RPE of 8.

Day	Target muscles	Exercises	Page #
Monday	Total body	Military press (3 sets @ 4-5RM)	75
		Barbell reverse-grip bent row (3 sets @ 4-5RM)	29
		Barbell chest press (3 sets @ 4-5RM)	47
		Deadlift (3 sets @ 4-5RM)	123
		Barbell back squat (3 sets @ 4-5RM)	119
Tuesday	Off		
Wednesday	Total body	Military press (3 sets @ 4-5RM)	75
		Barbell reverse-grip bent row (3 sets @ 4-5RM)	29
		Barbell chest press (3 sets @ 4-5RM)	47
		Deadlift (3 sets @ 4-5RM)	123
		Barbell back squat (3 sets @ 4-5RM)	119
Thursday	Off		
Friday	Total body	Military press (3 sets @ 4-5RM)	75
		Barbell reverse-grip bent row (3 sets @ 4-5RM)	29
		Barbell chest press (3 sets @ 4-5RM)	47
		Deadlift (3 sets @ 4-5RM)	123
		Barbell back squat (3 sets @ 4-5RM)	119
Saturday	Off		
Sunday	Off		

Table 7.3 Strength Phase Week 2: Block 1 Microcycle 2

Perform these exercises at an RPE of 9.

Day	Target muscles	Exercises	Page #
Monday	Total body	Military press (3 sets @ 2-3RM)	75
		Barbell reverse-grip bent row (3 sets @ 2-3RM)	29
		Barbell chest press (3 sets @ 2-3RM)	47
		Deadlift (3 sets @ 2-3RM)	123
		Barbell back squat (3 sets @ 2-3RM)	119
Tuesday	Off		
Wednesday	Total body	Military press (3 sets @ 2-3RM)	75
		Barbell reverse-grip bent row (3 sets @ 2-3RM)	29
		Barbell chest press (3 sets @ 2-3RM)	47
		Deadlift (3 sets @ 2-3RM)	123
		Barbell back squat (3 sets @ 2-3RM)	119
Thursday	Off		
Friday	Total body	Military press (3 sets @ 2-3RM)	75
		Barbell reverse-grip bent row (3 sets @ 2-3RM)	29
		Barbell chest press (3 sets @ 2-3RM)	47
		Deadlift (3 sets @ 2-3RM)	123
		Barbell back squat (3 sets @ 2-3RM)	119
Saturday	Off		
Sunday	Off		

Table 7.4 Strength Phase Week 3: Block 1 Microcycle 3

Perform the first set of exercises at an RPE of 8, perform the second set at an RPE of 9, and take the final maximal set to the point of concentric muscle failure.

Day	Target muscles	Exercises	Page #
Monday	Total body	Military press (3 sets @ 5RM, 3RM, 1RM)	75
		Barbell reverse-grip bent row (3 sets @ 5RM, 3RM, 1RM)	29
		Barbell chest press (3 sets @ 5RM, 3RM, 1RM)	47
		Deadlift (3 sets @ 5RM, 3RM, 1RM)	123
		Barbell back squat (3 sets @ 5RM, 3RM, 1RM)	119
Tuesday	Off		
Wednesday	Total body	Military press (3 sets @ 5RM, 3RM, 1RM)	75
		Barbell reverse-grip bent row (3 sets @ 5RM, 3RM, 1RM)	29
		Barbell chest press (3 sets @ 5RM, 3RM, 1RM)	47
		Deadlift (3 sets @ 5RM, 3RM, 1RM)	123
		Barbell back squat (3 sets @ 5RM, 3RM, 1RM)	119
Thursday	Off		
Friday	Total body	Military press (3 sets @ 5RM, 3RM, 1RM)	75
		Barbell reverse-grip bent row (3 sets @ 5RM, 3RM, 1RM)	29
		Barbell chest press (3 sets @ 5RM, 3RM, 1RM)	47
		Deadlift (3 sets @ 5RM, 3RM, 1RM)	123
		Barbell back squat (3 sets @ 5RM, 3RM, 1RM)	119
Saturday	Off		
Sunday	Off		

Table 7.5 Strength Phase Week 4: Block 1 Microcycle 4

Perform these exercises at an RPE of 7.

Day	Target muscles	Exercises	Page #
Monday	Total body	Dumbbell incline fly (3 sets @ 15-20RM)	52
		Lat pull-down (3 sets @ 15-20RM)	38
		Barbell upright row (3 sets @15-20 RM)	85
		Bulgarian squat (3 sets @ 15-20RM)	121
		Lying leg curl (3 sets @ 15-20RM)	133
		Machine standing calf raise (3 sets @ 15-20RM)	138
		Plank (3 sets @ 30 sec static hold)	64
Tuesday	Off		
Wednesday	Off		
Thursday	Total body	Cable fly (3 sets @ 15-20RM)	54
		Cable seated row (3 sets @ 15-20RM)	33
		Dumbbell lateral raise (3 sets @ 15-20RM)	78
		Dumbbell reverse lunge (3 sets @ 15-20RM)	115
		Machine seated leg curl (3 sets @ 15-20RM)	135
		Toe press (3 sets @ 15-20RM)	136
		Side bridge (3 sets @ 30 sec static hold)	65
Friday	Off		
Saturday	Off		
Sunday	Off		

Table 7.6   Strength Phase Week 5: Block 2 Microcycle 1

Perform these exercises at an RPE of 7 to 8.

Day	Target muscles	Exercises	Page #
Monday	Upper body	Military press (3 sets @ 4-5RM)	75
		Dumbbell lateral raise (3 sets @ 6-8RM)	78
		Barbell reverse-grip bent row (3 sets @ 4-5RM)	29
		Lat pull-down (3 sets @ 6-8RM)	38
		Barbell chest press (3 sets @ 4-5RM)	47
		Dumbbell incline fly (3 sets @ 6-8RM)	52
Tuesday	Lower body	Deadlift (3 sets @ 4-5RM)	123
		Barbell back squat (3 sets @ 4-5RM)	119
		Good morning (3 sets @ 6-8RM)	124
		Lying leg curl (3 sets @ 6-8RM)	133
		Machine standing calf raise (3 sets @ 6-8RM)	138
Wednesday	Off		
Thursday	Upper body	Military press (3 sets @ 4-5RM)	75
		Dumbbell lateral raise (3 sets @ 6-8RM)	78
		Barbell reverse-grip bent row (3 sets @ 4-5RM)	29
		Chin-up (3 sets @ 6-8RM)	36
		Barbell chest press (3 sets @ 4-5RM)	47
		Cable fly (3 sets @ 6-8RM)	54
Friday	Lower body	Deadlift (3 sets @ 4-5RM)	123
		Barbell back squat (3 sets @ 4-5RM)	119
		Barbell stiff-legged deadlift (3 sets @ 6-8RM)	127
		Machine seated leg curl (3 sets @ 6-8RM)	135
		Toe press (3 sets @ 6-8RM)	136
Saturday	Off		
Sunday	Off		

Table 7.7 Strength Phase Week 6: Block 2 Microcycle 2

Perform these exercises at an RPE of 8 to 9.

Day	Target muscles	Exercises	Page #
Monday	Upper body	Military press (3 sets @ 2-3RM)	75
		Dumbbell lateral raise (3 sets @ 6-8RM)	78
		Barbell reverse-grip bent row (3 sets @ 2-3RM)	29
		Lat pull-down (3 sets @ 6-8RM)	38
		Barbell chest press (3 sets @ 2-3RM)	47
		Dumbbell incline fly (3 sets @ 6-8RM)	52
Tuesday	Lower body	Deadlift (3 sets @ 2-3RM)	123
		Barbell back squat (3 sets @ 2-3RM)	119
		Good morning (3 sets @ 6-8RM)	124
		Lying leg curl (3 sets @ 6-8RM)	133
		Machine standing calf raise (3 sets @ 6-8RM)	138
Wednesday	Off		
Thursday	Upper body	Military press (3 sets @ 2-3RM)	75
		Dumbbell lateral raise (3 sets @ 6-8RM)	78
		Barbell reverse-grip bent row (3 sets @ 2-3RM)	29
		Chin-up (3 sets @ 6-8RM)	36
		Barbell chest press (3 sets @ 2-3RM)	47
		Cable fly (3 sets @ 6-8RM)	54
Friday	Lower body	Deadlift (3 sets @ 2-3RM)	123
		Barbell back squat (3 sets @ 2-3RM)	119
		Barbell stiff-legged deadlift (3 sets @ 6-8RM)	127
		Machine seated leg curl (3 sets @ 6-8RM)	135
		Toe press (3 sets @ 6-8RM)	136
Saturday	Off		
Sunday	Off		

Table 7.8   Strength Phase Week 7: Block 2 Microcycle 3

On the structural sets the first set (i.e., 4-5RM) should be performed at an RPE of 8, the second set (i.e., 2-3RM) should be performed at an RPE of 9, and the final maximal set (i.e., 1RM) should be taken to the point of concentric muscle failure. For assistance exercises, maintain an RM of 6 to 8 for all sets. Perform these exercises at an RPE of approximately 8 to 9.

Day	Target muscles	Exercises	Page #
Monday	Upper body	Military press (3 sets @ 5RM, 3RM, 1RM)	75
		Dumbbell lateral raise (3 sets @ 6-8RM)	78
		Barbell reverse-grip bent row (3 sets @ 5RM, 3RM, 1RM)	29
		Lat pull-down (3 sets @ 6-8RM)	38
		Barbell chest press (3 sets @ 5RM, 3RM, 1RM)	47
		Dumbbell incline fly (3 sets @ 6-8RM)	52
Tuesday	Lower body	Deadlift (3 sets @ 5RM, 3RM, 1RM)	123
		Barbell back squat (3 sets @ 5RM, 3RM, 1RM)	119
		Good morning (3 sets @ 6-8RM)	124
		Lying leg curl (3 sets @ 6-8RM)	133
		Machine standing calf raise (3 sets @ 6-8RM)	138
Wednesday	Off		
Thursday	Upper body	Military press (3 sets @ 5RM, 3RM, 1RM)	75
		Dumbbell lateral raise (3 sets @ 6-8RM)	78
		Barbell reverse-grip bent row (3 sets @ 5RM, 3RM, 1RM)	29
		Chin-up (3 sets @ 6-8RM)	36
		Barbell chest press (3 sets @ 5RM, 3RM, 1RM)	47
		Cable fly (3 sets @ 6-8RM)	54
Friday	Lower body	Deadlift (3 sets @ 5RM, 3RM, 1RM)	123
		Barbell back squat (3 sets @ 5RM, 3RM, 1RM)	119
		Barbell stiff-legged deadlift (3 sets @ 6-8RM)	127
		Machine seated leg curl (3 sets @ 6-8RM)	135
		Toe press (3 sets @ 6-8RM)	136
Saturday	Off		
Sunday	Off		

Table 7.9 Strength Phase Week 8: Block 2 Microcycle 4

Perform these exercises at an RPE of about 7.

Day	Target muscles	Exercises	Page #
Monday	Total body	Dumbbell incline fly (3 sets @ 15-20RM)	52
		Lat pull-down (3 sets @ 15-20RM)	38
		Barbell upright row (3 sets @ 15-20RM)	85
		Bulgarian squat (3 sets @ 15-20RM)	121
		Lying leg curl (3 sets @ 15-20RM)	133
		Machine standing calf raise (3 sets @ 15-20RM)	138
		Plank (3 sets @ 30 sec static hold)	64
Tuesday	Off		
Wednesday	Off		
Thursday	Total body	Cable fly (3 sets @ 15-20RM)	54
		Cable seated row (3 sets @ 15-20RM)	33
		Dumbbell lateral raise (3 sets @ 15-20RM)	78
		Dumbbell reverse lunge (3 sets @ 15-20RM)	115
		Machine seated leg curl (3 sets @ 15-20RM)	135
		Toe press (3 sets @ 15-20RM)	136
		Side bridge (3 sets @ 30 sec static hold)	65
Friday	Off		
Saturday	Off		
Sunday	Off		

CHAPTER 8

MAX Metabolic Phase

The MAX metabolic phase is a preparatory phase that conditions your body for hypertrophy training. The goal is to optimize training efficiency by packing more exercise into less time. This is accomplished by combining high repetitions (15-20) with short rest intervals (30 seconds or less). Rest intervals progressively decrease over the course of the cycle to bring about the desired metabolic adaptations.

On the surface, metabolic training might seem counterintuitive to building muscle. After all, we've already established that high-rep training doesn't generate a whole lot of muscle tension, and given that tension is the main driving force for protein synthesis, it stands to reason that using light weights is not going to pack on much muscle. Although this is certainly true, consider the bigger picture. Over the long term, a properly structured metabolic-training cycle can help set the stage for greater muscle growth in several ways.

First and foremost, metabolic training increases your lactate threshold—the point at which lactic acid begins to rapidly accumulate in working muscles. From a muscle-building standpoint, lactic acid is a double-edged sword. On one hand, it's involved in the acute anabolic hormonal response to training, cell swelling, and other potentially important aspects of muscle development. On the other hand, excessive buildup of lactic acid can interfere with muscle contraction, thus reducing the number of reps you can perform. Here's where metabolic training comes to the rescue. Adaptations associated with metabolic training include an increase in the number of capillaries (tiny blood vessels that facilitate the exchange of nutrients and metabolic waste) and an improved muscle-buffering capacity, both of which help delay lactic buildup. The upshot is that you're able to maintain greater time under tension without compromising the hypertrophy-related benefits of lactate accumulation. In addition, you develop a greater tolerance for higher volumes of work—an important component of maximizing hypertrophy.

Metabolic training also improves glycogen storage capacity. Glycogen is the term for stored carbohydrate. The majority of glycogen is stored in muscle tissue, and the balance is deposited in liver cells. Here's the kicker: Each gram of stored glycogen attracts three grams of water into the muscle. Increase muscle glycogen stores and you increase your ability to get a better pump during training. Recall that the pump is indicative of cellular hydration, which has been shown to enhance protein synthesis and decrease protein breakdown—a win–win for increasing lean muscle.

In addition, metabolic training enhances your recovery ability. As mentioned, training in a metabolic fashion increases the network of capillaries that deliver nutrients (such as oxygen, hormones, amino acids, and so on) to body tissues. A greater capillary density allows for greater nutrient transfer to your muscles. This facilitates better recovery after a long workout in that it supplies damaged muscles with the necessary materials for repair and regeneration.

Finally, metabolic training helps fully stimulate the growth of slow-twitch muscle fibers. Although slow-twitch fibers are often dismissed as irrelevant from a muscle-building standpoint, don't discount their importance to overall muscle development. Superior slow-twitch fiber hypertrophy is a primary reason bodybuilders display greater muscularity compared with powerlifters. To maximize muscle size, it is necessary to stimulate the full spectrum of fibers, including slow-twitch fibers.

Before you take this to mean that including extended cycles of metabolic training in a hypertrophy program is beneficial, remember that this type of training is intended to set the stage for muscle development, not to directly build appreciable muscle. In fact, prolonged periods of metabolic training can negatively affect force production and fast-twitch muscle fiber size. Thus, limit metabolic cycles to short time periods to avoid any detrimental effect on your physique.

Moreover, the weights used in this phase are comparatively light, but that doesn't mean that the workouts will be a walk in the park. Quite the contrary. Metabolic training can be even more physically demanding than heavy-weight training. Pushing past the intense burn that builds up during a high-rep set requires a high tolerance for discomfort and lots of resolve. It's definitely not for the weak of mind!

PROGRAM PROTOCOL

The MAX metabolic phase of the MAX Muscle Plan is a four-week, low-intensity mesocycle consisting of a single training block. It's long enough to promote desired metabolic adaptations without compromising muscle strength and size. Three metabolic training strategies are used over the course of the mesocycle. Here is an overview of each strategy.

1. **Straight-set metabolic training.** Straight-set metabolic training is similar to traditional strength training: You perform a given number of sets for an exercise, proceed to the next exercise for a given number of sets (for our purposes you perform three sets), and so on until you've completed the routine. Simple, right? The unique aspect of straight-set metabolic training is that repetitions are maintained in the high range (15-20 reps per set) and rest intervals are very brief (30 seconds between sets). This results in high amounts of metabolic stress that causes an intense sensation, or burn, in the working muscles. Because rest periods are short, your body won't have sufficient time to recover. Thus, you'll need to progressively decrease the amount of weight used in the second and third sets of an exercise to maintain the target rep range. Don't be concerned. Remember, the goal of metabolic training is to increase your lactate threshold and promote slow-twitch fiber hypertrophy; the load is of secondary consequence.

2. **Paired-set training.** A superset is two exercises performed in succession without rest. From a metabolic standpoint, one of the best supersetting methods is paired-set training. This technique supersets exercises that share an agonist–antagonist relationship, meaning that when one muscle contracts, the muscle on the opposing side of the body relaxes. Although paired-set training often focuses on opposing muscle groups (e.g., back and chest, biceps and triceps, quads and hamstrings), you'll base exercising pairings on opposing joint actions such as flexion–extension and abduction–adduction. Plantarflexion (e.g., calf raises) and spinal flexion (e.g., crunches) are not paired because their antagonist movements (dorsiflexion and spinal hyperextension, respectively) have little relevance to hypertrophy-oriented routines.

   To ensure optimal efficiency, set up exercise stations in advance so that you are able to move quickly between exercises. You'll perform a set of the first exercise, proceed directly to the second movement as quickly as possible, rest for approximately 30 seconds, and then repeat for two additional supersets. Then move on to the next agonist–antagonist pairing and so on until you complete all paired sets.

3. **Circuit training.** As opposed to straight-set training, circuit training requires that you move from one exercise to the next with minimal rest (ideally less than 10 seconds). In essence, you perform one giant set of multiple exercises for different muscle groups. To facilitate your ability to transition swiftly between movements, set up in advance a series of exercise stations that work muscles in a push–pull fashion. Start with upper-body exercises and proceed to movements for the lower body; perform abdominal exercises last in the sequence (i.e., chest, back, shoulders, biceps, triceps, quads, hamstrings, calves, abdomen). After

finishing the circuit, go back to the first exercise and perform two additional circuits in the same expeditious fashion.

You'll perform three sets per muscle group and follow a total-body routine that works all the major muscles during each session. The key to optimizing results is to train at maximal or near-maximal levels of effort. Take sets to the point of muscle failure, or at least close to it (equal to an RPE of 9 or 10). It's important to feel the burn as you reach the last few reps. This burning sensation indicates that you're accumulating metabolites. If you aren't sufficiently pushing yourself to complete each set, the metabolic effect will be compromised.

Multijoint exercises are incorporated into the routine whenever possible. Research shows that the metabolic cost of an exercise is directly related to the amount of muscle worked (Farinatt, Castinheiras, and Neto 2011). In other words, involve more muscle and you increase metabolic work. Thus, squats, rows, presses, and the like are used to work the muscles of the torso and thighs; single-joint movements are reserved for the muscles of the arms and calves.

To condition as many muscle fibers as possible, you'll perform a greater variety of exercises during this phase than during the MAX strength phase. Considering that you will perform sets with limited rest, this can be a challenge if you work out in a crowded gym. In this case, simply substitute a comparable exercise that targets similar muscles. Minimizing rest intervals is far and away the most important objective. If you have to sacrifice some variety to achieve greater expediency, so be it.

Perform repetitions at a moderately fast tempo, particularly on the concentric portion of the movement. Aim to perform concentric lifts as explosively as possible without getting sloppy with your technique. On the other hand, perform eccentric reps somewhat slower, making sure that working muscles resist gravitational pull on the negative phase of each rep. Eccentric exercise has a significant effect on resistance training-induced metabolic stress. If weights are not lowered under control, results suffer. An eccentric cadence of approximately two to three seconds is optimal.

PROGRAM SPECIFICS

The MAX metabolic phase consists of a single training block made up of four one-week microcycles. Rest intervals between sets progressively decrease over the first three microcycles and RPE increases to generate increased metabolic stress; intensity and volume stay relatively constant. The final week is a low-volume unloading cycle that will restore and rejuvenate. Here are the particulars for each microcycle.

The first microcycle (week 1 of the mesocycle) incorporates straight-set metabolic training. Carry out the first two sets at near-maximal intensity (equal to an RPE of 9). Take the last set of each exercise to the point of concentric muscle failure. Aim for 15 to 20 reps per set. If you can't perform at least 15 reps, lighten the weight; if you can perform more than 20 reps, increase the weight. Rest about 30 seconds between sets—just long enough to catch your breath. After finishing all three sets of an exercise, move quickly to the next exercise, taking no more than about 30 seconds between movements.

The second microcycle (week 2) incorporates reciprocal supersets. Carry out the first two sets at near-maximal intensity (equal to an RPE of 9). Take the last set of each exercise to the point of concentric muscle failure. Aim for 15 to 20 reps per set. If you can't perform at least 15 reps, lighten the weight; if you can perform more than 20 reps, increase the weight. Take approximately 30 seconds of rest between each superset. After finishing all three sets of a superset combo, move quickly to the next superset, taking no more than 30 seconds between movements.

The third microcycle (week 3) incorporates circuit training. Take all sets to the point of concentric muscle failure. Aim for 15 to 20 reps per set. If you can't perform at least 15 reps, lighten the weight; if you can perform more than 20 reps, increase the weight. Move from one exercise to the next as quickly as possible—keep rest to an absolute minimum. After finishing the entire circuit, repeat the process two more times, again resting as little as possible.

The fourth microcycle (week 4) is an unloading phase. You'll train two days per week, allowing 72 hours between sessions (e.g., Monday and Thursday), and follow a total-body routine that works all the major muscle groups during each session. One exercise of three sets will be performed per muscle group. Intensity should be 15- to 20RM. Effort should equate to an RPE of about 7.

Table 8.1 summarizes the MAX metabolic phase protocol, and sample routines (tables 8.2 through 8.5) are provided on the subsequent pages. These routines should serve as a basic template for constructing your workouts. Modify specific exercises according to your individual needs and abilities.

Table 8.1 Summary of MAX Metabolic Protocol

Training variable	Protocol
Repetitions	15-20
Sets	3 per exercise
Rest interval	30 sec or less
Tempo	Concentric: explosive Eccentric: 2-3 sec
Frequency	3 days per week

Table 8.2   Metabolic Phase Week 1: Microcycle 1

Perform these exercises at an RPE of 9. Rest 30 seconds between sets.

Day	Target muscles	Exercises	Page #
Monday	Total body	Dumbbell incline press (3 sets @ 15-20RM)	43
		Dumbbell one-arm row (3 sets @ 15-20RM)	27
		Dumbbell shoulder press (3 sets @ 15-20RM)	76
		Dumbbell standing biceps curl (3 sets @ 15-20RM)	87
		Dumbbell overhead triceps extension (3 sets @ 15-20RM)	100
		Leg press (3 sets @ 15-20RM)	122
		Lying leg curl (3 sets @ 15-20RM)	133
		Machine standing calf raise (3 sets @ 15-20RM)	138
		Bicycle crunch (3 sets @ 15-20RM)	58
Tuesday	Off		
Wednesday	Total body	Barbell chest press (3 sets @ 15-20RM)	47
		Lat pull-down (3 sets @ 15-20RM)	38
		Barbell upright row (3 sets @ 15-20RM)	85
		Barbell curl (3 sets @ 15-20RM)	95
		Cable triceps press-down (3 sets @ 15-20RM)	107
		Barbell back squat (3 sets @ 15-20RM)	119
		Machine seated leg curl (3 sets @ 15-20RM)	135
		Machine seated calf raise (3 sets @ 15-20RM)	137
		Cable rope kneeling crunch (3 sets @ 15-20RM)	61
Thursday	Off		
Friday	Total body	Machine chest press (3 sets @ 15-20RM)	50
		Cable seated row (3 sets @ 15-20RM)	33
		Military press (3 sets @ 15-20RM)	75
		Cable curl (3 sets @ 15-20RM)	98
		Nosebreaker (3 sets @ 15-20RM)	102
		Walking lunge (3 sets @ 15-20RM)	112
		Barbell stiff-legged deadlift (3 sets @ 15-20RM)	127
		Toe press (3 sets @ 15-20RM)	136
		Roman chair side crunch (3 sets @ 15-20RM)	59
Saturday	Off		
Sunday	Off		

Table 8.3 Metabolic Phase Week 2: Microcycle 2

Perform these exercises at an RPE of 9. Rest 30 seconds between supersets.

Day	Target muscles	Exercises	Page #
Monday	Total body	Dumbbell chest press supersetted with cable seated row (3 sets @ 15-20RM)	45 and 33
		Military press supersetted with lat pull-down (3 sets @ 15-20RM)	75 and 38
		Barbell curl supersetted with triceps dip (3 sets @ 15-20RM)	95 and 108
		Leg press supersetted with machine seated leg curl (3 sets @ 15-20RM)	122 and 135
Tuesday	Off		
Wednesday	Total body	Barbell incline press supersetted with barbell reverse-grip bent row (3 sets @ 15-20RM)	46 and 29
		Dumbbell shoulder press supersetted with cross cable lat pull-down (3 sets @ 15-20RM)	76 and 42
		Dumbbell standing biceps curl supersetted with machine nosebreaker (3 sets @ 15-20RM)	87 and 103
		Barbell front squat supersetted with dumbbell stiff-legged deadlift (3 sets @ 15-20RM)	118 and 127
Thursday	Off		
Friday	Total body	Barbell decline press supersetted with dumbbell one-arm row (3 sets @ 15-20RM)	48 and 27
		Cable upright row supersetted with lat pull-down—V-bar variation (3 sets @ 15-20RM)	86 and 38
		Cable curl supersetted with cable triceps press-down (3 sets @ 15-20RM)	98 and 107
		Walking lunge supersetted with lying leg curl (3 sets @ 15-20RM)	112 and 133
Saturday	Off		
Sunday	Off		

Table 8.4   Metabolic Phase Week 3: Microcycle 3

Take each set to the point of concentric muscle failure. Rest as little as possible between supersets.

Day	Target muscles	Exercises	Page #
Monday	Total body	Dumbbell incline chest press (3 sets @ 15-20RM)	43
		Dumbbell one-arm row (3 sets @ 15-20RM)	27
		Dumbbell shoulder press (3 sets @ 15-20RM)	76
		Dumbbell standing biceps curl (3 sets @ 15-20RM)	87
		Dumbbell overhead triceps extension (3 sets @ 15-20RM)	100
		Leg press (3 sets @ 15-20RM)	122
		Lying leg curl (3 sets @ 15-20RM)	133
		Machine standing calf raise (3 sets @ 15-20RM)	138
		Bicycle crunch (3 sets @ 15-20RM)	58
Tuesday	Off		
Wednesday	Total body	Barbell chest press (3 sets @ 15-20RM)	47
		Lat pull-down (3 sets @ 15-20RM)	38
		Barbell upright row (3 sets @ 15-20RM)	85
		Barbell curl (3 sets @ 15-20RM)	95
		Cable triceps press-down (3 sets @ 15-20RM)	107
		Barbell back squat (3 sets @ 15-20RM)	119
		Machine seated leg curl (3 sets @ 15-20RM)	135
		Machine seated calf raise (3 sets @ 15-20RM)	137
		Cable rope kneeling crunch (3 sets @ 15-20RM)	61
Thursday	Off		
Friday	Total body	Machine chest press (3 sets @ 15-20RM)	50
		Cable seated row (3 sets @ 15-20RM)	33
		Military press (3 sets @ 15-20RM)	75
		Cable curl (3 sets @ 15-20RM)	98
		Nosebreaker (3 sets @ 15-20RM)	102
		Walking lunge (3 sets @ 15-20RM)	112
		Barbell stiff-legged deadlift (3 sets @ 15-20RM)	127
		Toe press (3 sets @ 15-20RM)	136
		Roman chair side crunch (3 sets @ 15-20RM)	59
Saturday	Off		
Sunday	Off		

Table 8.5 Metabolic Phase Week 4: Microcycle 4

Perform these exercises at an RPE of 7.

Day	Target muscles	Exercises	Page #
Monday	Total body	Dumbbell incline fly (3 sets @ 15-20RM)	52
		Lat pull-down (3 sets @ 15-20RM)	38
		Barbell upright row (3 sets @ 15-20RM)	85
		Bulgarian squat (3 sets @ 15-20RM)	121
		Lying leg curl (3 sets @ 15-20RM)	133
		Machine standing calf raise (3 sets @ 15-20RM)	138
		Plank (3 sets @ 30 sec static hold)	64
Tuesday	Off		
Wednesday	Off		
Thursday	Total body	Cable fly (3 sets @ 15-20RM)	54
		Cable seated row (3 sets @ 15-20RM)	33
		Dumbbell lateral raise (3 sets @ 15-20RM)	78
		Dumbbell reverse lunge (3 sets @ 15-20RM)	115
		Machine seated leg curl (3 sets @ 15-20RM)	135
		Toe press (3 sets @ 15-20RM)	136
		Side bridge (3 sets @ 30 sec static hold)	65
Friday	Off		
Saturday	Off		
Sunday	Off		

CHAPTER 9

MAX Muscle Phase

The MAX muscle phase is the culmination of the MAX Muscle Plan. As the name implies, this phase maximizes muscle development from both a quantitative (muscle size) and a qualitative (muscle symmetry) standpoint. You'll expend a lot of sweat and effort, but the results will be well worth it—guaranteed!

This phase capitalizes on the gains you achieved in the previous phases of the program. Specifically, the strength you gained in the MAX strength phase will facilitate your ability to handle heavier weights—and thus enhance levels of muscle tension—during hypertrophy training. What's more, the improved metabolic efficiency you achieved in the MAX metabolic phase will allow for increased time under tension for your muscles and heighten your capacity to tolerate greater volumes of work. In the muscle phase you'll take advantage of all these adaptations, leveraging them to reach your muscular potential.

PROGRAM PROTOCOL

The MAX muscle phase is a 12-week mesocycle made up of three training blocks followed by a recovery period. You'll use moderate-intensity loads (6-12RM) with moderate rest intervals (60-90 seconds between sets). This combination elicits an optimal mix of muscle tension and metabolic stress—a formula that is essential to maximizing muscle development.

You'll perform a total of 25 to 30 sets per session and do multiple sets for each exercise. You'll work larger muscle groups (such as the quads, glutes, and back) with a high training volume. Conversely, the muscles of the arms and calves are the target of fewer total direct sets because they are smaller and they function as secondary muscle movers in many mulitjoint exercises.

Training frequency progressively increases over the course of the meso-cycle, which culminates with a shock phase that will bring about short-term overreaching (see Table 9.1 for a schedule). Reduced-frequency unloading phases are interspersed throughout the mesocycle to ensure adequate recu-peration. In general, the full effects of supercompensation will manifest one

Table 9.1 Training Frequency Schedule

Block	Microcycle	Training frequency	Days	Regions targeted
1	1-3	3 days per week	Monday Wednesday Friday	Chest, shoulders, triceps Legs Back, biceps, abdomen
	4	2 days per week (unloading)	Monday, Thursday	Total body
2	1-3	4 days per week	Monday, Thursday Tuesday, Friday	Upper body Lower body
	4	2 days per week (unloading)	Monday, Thursday	Total body
3	1-2	6 days per week	Monday, Friday Tuesday, Saturday Wednesday, Sunday	Back, chest, abdomen Legs Shoulders, arms
		Active recovery		Light aerobic exercise

to two weeks after you complete an overreaching microcycle. This means that you should realize optimal muscle gains sometime during the active recovery microcycle.

Exercises rotate from one workout to the next to ensure the complete stimulation of the full spectrum of muscle fibers. I have carefully selected the exercises in the sample routines to work different areas of the target muscles in each training session. In effect, the exercises complement one another; overlap between movements is minimal. To ensure that you work each muscle to its full extent, a mix of modalities (free weights, machines, and cables) is used over the course of the mesocycle.

To increase the growth response, several special training techniques are integrated into this phase. The use of these techniques is limited to a select few sets throughout the training cycle because the fatiguing nature of these techniques increases the potential for overtraining. Here is an overview of the special techniques that you'll use in this phase.

Drop Sets

Drop sets, also known as strip sets or descending sets, involve performing a set to muscle failure with a given load and then immediately reducing the load and continuing to train until subsequent failure. This technique enhances muscle fiber fatigue and metabolic stress. Aim to strip off the weights as quickly as possible; resting more than a few seconds between drop sets diminishes the beneficial effects of the technique. You can perform multiple drops in the same set to elicit even greater fatigue and stress.

Variety

For the MAX muscle phase, I have endeavored to change up the exercises from one workout to the next using a multi-angled, multi-planar, multi-modality approach. As discussed previously, performing an assortment of moves helps to stimulate all of the fibers in your major muscles to elicit maximal muscle growth and symmetry. Is all this variety absolutely essential? No. My intention here was simply to show the potential for incorporating different movements into your routine, not to suggest that every workout must be different from the previous one. That said, you should strive to change the exercises on a regular basis. There is no hard and fast rule as to how often such changes should be implemented, but a good rule of thumb is to switch things up at least every few weeks. Remember, variety is the spice of muscle development!

Paired Sets

Recall that we used paired-set training in the MAX metabolic phase of the program to take advantage of the high metabolite buildup associated with supersetting. Paired-set training also can help increase muscle development—provided that intensity and rest intervals correspond to a hypertrophy range. As opposed to same-muscle supersets, reciprocal supersets do not cause much of a reduction in strength. In fact, contracting an antagonist muscle actually can increase force output during subsequent contractions of the agonist. This is presumably the result of reduced antagonist inhibition and possibly stored elastic energy in the muscle–tendon complex. As you know by now, greater muscle tension generated by the agonist means greater increases in muscle growth, particularly in the presence of high amounts of metabolic stress. To take advantage of this effect, do the following. Set up agonist–antagonist exercise stations so that you are able to move quickly between movements. Perform a set of the first exercise, proceed directly to the second movement, rest for approximately 30 seconds, and then repeat for two additional super-sets. Then move on to the next agonist–antagonist pairing and so on until you have completed all paired sets.

Heavy Negatives

Heavy negatives involve performing eccentric contractions at a weight greater than your concentric 1RM. Studies show that including heavy negatives in a routine can magnify the growth response, likely as a result of a combination of factors, including greater inroading, muscle damage, and metabolic stress (Schoenfeld 2011). The protocol for the technique is as follows. Load the bar with a weight that is approximately 25 percent heavier than your 1RM for a given exercise. For example, if your maximum bench press is 200 pounds (90.7 kg), use 250 pounds (113.4 kg). Perform an eccentric repetition at a tempo of approximately two to three seconds, making sure to lower the weights in a controlled fashion. When you reach the bottom portion of the lift, have a spotter help you raise the weight back to the start position. Aim for three to four reps per set. Do not attempt this technique without using a spotter! If a spotter is not available, simply substitute drop sets.

PROGRAM SPECIFICS

As noted, the MAX muscle phase mesocycle segments training into three blocks that consist of four one-week microcycles. Training volume progressively increases each block so that you achieve the high volume necessary to maximize growth without risking overtraining. In effect, each block builds on the results achieved in the previous block. Intensity varies using a step-loading model in which unloading cycles are interspersed at regular intervals to promote optimal recovery.

Here are the particulars of each block.

Block 1

Block 1 is made up of four one-week microcycles. During the first three microcycles, you'll train on three nonconsecutive days per week (e.g., Monday, Wednesday, and Friday). Training incorporates a three-day push–pull split: You'll work the chest, shoulders, and triceps on day 1; the lower-body musculature on day 2; and the back, biceps, and abdomen on day 3. You'll perform three to four sets of two to four exercises per muscle group. Intensity is carried out using the following step-loading progression.

The first microcycle in block 1 (week 1 of the mesocycle) targets an intensity corresponding to 10- to 12RM. Your level of effort should correspond to an RPE of 8 to 9 on the initial sets of each exercise, and you should take the last set to the point of concentric muscle failure (RPE of 10).

The second microcycle in block 1 (week 2) targets an intensity corresponding to 8- to 10RM. Your level of effort should correspond to an RPE of 8 to 9 on the initial sets of each exercise, and you should take the last set to the point of concentric muscle failure (RPE of 10) and perform double drop sets.

The third microcycle in block 1 (week 3) targets an intensity corresponding to 6- to 8RM. Take all sets to the point of concentric muscle failure (RPE of 10). After finishing all sets for the chest, back, and thighs, you'll perform an additional set of heavy negatives for that muscle group.

The fourth microcycle in block 1 (week 4) is an unloading phase. You'll train two days per week, allowing 72 hours between sessions (e.g., Monday and Thursday), and follow a total-body routine that works all the major muscle groups during each session. You'll perform one exercise of three sets per muscle group. Intensity will be 15- to 20RM. Sets should not be overly challenging. Aim for an RPE of 7 or so. If you struggle on the last few reps, lighten the weight!

Block 2

Block 2 is made up of four one-week microcycles. During the first three microcycles, you'll train four days per week using a sequence of either two on, one off, two on, two off (e.g., Monday, Tuesday, Thursday, and Friday) or two on, one off, one on, one off, one on, one off (e.g., Monday, Tuesday, Thursday, and Saturday). Training incorporates a two-day split: you'll work the upper body on day 1 and the lower body on day 2. The abdomen is included on the lower-body days. You'll perform three to four sets of one to two exercises per muscle group. Intensity is carried out using the following step-loading progression.

The first microcycle in block 2 (week 5 of the mesocycle) targets an intensity corresponding to 10- to 12RM. Your level of effort should correspond to an RPE of 8 to 9 on the initial sets of each exercise, and you should take the last set to the point of concentric muscle failure (RPE of 10).

The second microcycle in block 2 (week 6) targets an intensity corresponding to 8- to 10RM. Your level of effort should correspond to an RPE of 8 to 9 on the initial sets of each exercise, and you should take the last set to the point of concentric muscle failure (RPE of 10) and perform double drop sets.

The third microcycle in block 2 (week 7) targets an intensity corresponding to 6- to 8RM. Take all sets to the point of concentric muscle failure (RPE of 10). After completing all sets for the chest, back, and thighs, you'll perform an additional set of heavy negatives for that muscle group.

The fourth microcycle in block 2 (week 8) is an unloading phase. You'll train two days per week, allowing 72 hours between sessions (e.g., Monday and Thursday), and follow a total-body routine that works all the major muscle groups during each session. You'll perform one exercise of three sets per muscle group. Intensity will be 15- to 20RM. Sets should not be overly challenging. As with the previous unloading phase, aim for an RPE of about 7.

Block 3

Block 3 is made up of two one-week microcycles. During each of the two microcycles, you'll train six days per week using a sequence of three on, one off, three on (i.e., Monday, Tuesday, Wednesday, Friday, Saturday, and

Sunday). Training incorporates a three-day, agonist–antagonist split: You'll work the back, chest, and abdomen on day 1; the lower-body musculature on day 2; and the shoulders and arms on day 3. You'll perform three to four sets of two to four exercises per muscle group. Intensity is carried out using the following progression.

The first microcycle (week 9) targets an intensity corresponding to 10- to 12RM. Take all sets to the point of concentric muscle failure (RPE of 10). You'll perform supersets for agonist–antagonist muscle groups.

The second microcycle (week 10) targets an intensity corresponding to 6- to 8RM. Take all sets to the point of concentric muscle failure (RPE of 10). You'll perform double drop sets on the last set of each exercise.

Following block 3 is an active recovery period that lasts one to two weeks. This period allows for optimal restoration of your body's resources and helps prevent the potential for overtraining. During this time, perform only light, continuous aerobic exercise at an RPE of 5 on the 1 to 10 scale for 30 to 40 minutes most days of the week. Exercise modalities should incorporate both upper- and lower-body musculature (e.g., elliptical trainers, cross-country ski trainers, jumping jacks) to enhance blood flow throughout the body. Perform no resistance training during this time.

Table 9.2 summarizes the MAX muscle phase protocol, and sample routines (tables 9.3 through 9.12) are provided on the subsequent pages. These routines should serve as a basic template for constructing your workouts. Modify specific exercises according to your individual needs and abilities.

Table 9.2 Summary of MAX Muscle Protocol

Training variable	Protocol
Repetitions	6-12
Sets	2-4 per exercise
Rest interval	60-90 sec
Tempo	Concentric: explosive Eccentric: 2-3 sec
Frequency	3-6 days per week

Table 9.3 Muscle Phase Week 1: Block 1 Microcycle 1

Perform initial sets at an RPE of 8 to 9 and take the last set to the point of concentric muscle failure.

Day	Target muscles	Exercises	Page #
Monday	Chest, shoulders, triceps	Barbell incline press (4 sets @ 10-12RM)	46
		Dumbbell chest press (4 sets @ 10-12RM)	45
		Pec deck fly (3 sets @ 10-12RM)	53
		Military press (4 sets @ 10-12RM)	75
		Dumbbell lateral raise (3 sets @ 10-12RM)	78
		Machine rear delt fly (3 sets @ 10-12RM)	82
		Dumbbell overhead triceps extension (3 sets @ 10-12RM)	100
		Nosebreaker (2 sets @ 10-12RM)	102
		Machine triceps dip (2 sets @ 10-12RM)	109
Tuesday	Off		
Wednesday	Legs	Barbell back squat (4 sets @ 10-12RM)	119
		Dumbbell reverse lunge (4 sets @ 10-12RM)	115
		Leg extension (3 sets @ 10-12RM)	131
		Barbell stiff-legged deadlift (4 sets @ 10-12RM)	126
		Lying leg curl (4 sets @ 10-12RM)	133
		Machine seated calf raise (4 sets @ 10-12RM)	137
		Machine standing calf raise (3 sets @ 10-12RM)	138
Thursday	Off		
Friday	Back, biceps, abdomen	Lat pull-down (4 sets @ 10-12RM)	38
		Cable seated row (4 sets @ 10-12RM)	33
		Dumbbell pullover (4 sets @ 10-12RM)	26
		Barbell curl (3 sets @ 10-12RM)	95
		Cable rope hammer curl (2 sets @ 10-12RM)	97
		Concentration curl (2 sets @ 10-12RM)	93
		Stability ball abdominal crunch (4 sets @ 10-12RM)	60
		Reverse crunch (3 sets @ 10-12RM)	57
		Russian twist (3 sets @ 10-12RM)	67
Saturday	Off		
Sunday	Off		

Table 9.4 Muscle Phase Week 2: Block 1 Microcycle 2

Perform initial sets at an RPE of 8 to 9 and take the last set to the point of concentric muscle failure.

Day	Target muscles	Exercises	Page #
Monday	Chest, shoulders, triceps	Dumbbell incline press (4 sets @ 8-10RM)	43
		Barbell decline press (4 sets @ 8-10RM)	48
		Dumbbell flat fly (3 sets @ 8-10RM)	51
		Dumbbell shoulder press (4 sets @ 8-10RM)	76
		Cable upright row (4 sets @ 8-10RM)	86
		Dumbbell bent reverse fly (3 sets @ 8-10RM)	81
		Cable rope overhead triceps extension (3 sets @ 8-10RM)	101
		Cable triceps press-down (2 sets @ 8-10RM)	107
		Triceps dip (2 sets @ 8-10RM)	108
Tuesday	Off		
Wednesday	Legs	Barbell front squat (4 sets @ 8-10RM)	118
		Dumbbell step-up (4 sets @ 8-10RM)	117
		Sissy squat (3 sets @ 8-10RM)	125
		Good morning (4 sets @ 8-10RM)	124
		Machine seated leg curl (4 sets @ 8-10RM)	135
		Toe press (4 sets @ 8-10RM)	136
		Machine seated calf raise (3 sets @ 8-10RM)	137
Thursday	Off		
Friday	Back, biceps, abdomen	Cross cable lat pull-down (4 sets @ 8-10RM)	42
		Dumbbell one-arm row (4 sets @ 8-10RM)	27
		Cable straight-arm lat pull-down (3 sets @ 8-10RM)	41
		Dumbbell incline biceps curl (4 sets @ 8-10RM)	88
		Barbell preacher curl (3 sets @ 8-10RM)	91
		Hanging knee raise (4 sets @ 8-10RM)	66
		Dumbbell side bend (3 sets @ 8-10RM)	68
		Cable wood chop (3 sets @ 8-10RM)	70
Saturday	Off		
Sunday	Off		

Table 9.5 Muscle Phase Week 3: Block 1 Microcycle 3

Perform all sets to the point of concentric muscle failure.

Day	Target muscles	Exercises	Page #
Monday	Chest, shoulders, triceps	Machine chest press (4 sets @ 6-8RM)	50
		Dumbbell incline press (4 sets @ 6-8RM)	43
		Cable fly (3 sets @ 6-8RM)	54
		Arnold press (4 sets @ 6-8RM)	74
		Machine lateral raise (3 sets @ 6-8RM)	79
		Cable reverse fly (3 sets @ 6-8RM)	83
		Machine nosebreaker (3 sets @ 6-8RM)	103
		Dumbbell triceps kickback (2 sets @ 6-8RM)	104
		Cable triceps kickback (2 sets @ 6-8RM)	105
Tuesday	Off		
Wednesday	Legs	Leg press (4 sets @ 6-8RM)	122
		Dumbbell lunge (4 sets @ 6-8RM)	114
		One-leg extension (3 sets @ 6-8RM)	132
		Reverse hyperextension (4 sets @ 6-8RM)	130
		Machine kneeling leg curl (4 sets @ 6-8RM)	134
		Machine seated calf raise (4 sets @ 6-8RM)	137
		Machine standing calf raise (4 sets @ 6-8RM)	138
Thursday	Off		
Friday	Back, biceps, abdomen	Chin-up (4 sets @ 6-8RM)	36
		Machine wide-grip seated row (4 sets @ 6-8RM)	32
		Cable one-arm standing low row (4 sets @ 6-8RM)	35
		Cable one-arm curl (3 sets @ 6-8RM)	99
		Dumbbell standing hammer curl (2 sets @ 6-8RM)	94
		Machine preacher curl (2 sets @ 6-8RM)	92
		Toe touch (4 sets @ 6-8RM)	63
		Cable side bend (3 sets @ 6-8RM)	69
		Side bridge (3 sets @ 6-8RM)	65
Saturday	Off		
Sunday	Off		

Table 9.6 Muscle Phase Week 4: Block 1 Microcycle 4

Perform these exercises at an RPE of 7.

Day	Target muscles	Exercises	Page #
Monday	Total body	Barbell incline press (3 sets @ 15-20RM)	46
		Lat pull-down (3 sets @ 15-20RM)	38
		Barbell upright row (3 sets @ 15-20RM)	85
		Barbell curl (3 sets @ 15-20RM)	95
		Nosebreaker (3 sets @ 15-20RM)	102
		Barbell back squat (3 sets @ 15-20RM)	119
		Lying leg curl (3 sets @ 15-20RM)	133
		Machine standing calf raise (3 sets @ 15-20RM)	138
		Plank (3 sets @ 30 sec static hold)	64
Tuesday	Off		
Wednesday	Off		
Thursday	Total body	Dumbbell chest press (3 sets @ 15-20RM)	45
		Barbell overhand bent row (3 sets @ 15-20RM)	30
		Military press (3 sets @ 15-20RM)	75
		Dumbbell preacher curl (3 sets @ 15-20RM)	90
		Cable triceps press-down (3 sets @ 15-20RM)	107
		Dumbbell reverse lunge (3 sets @ 15-20RM)	115
		Cable glute kickback (3 sets @ 15-20RM)	128
		Toe press (3 sets @ 15-20RM)	136
		Side bridge (3 sets @ 30 sec static hold)	65
Friday	Off		
Saturday	Off		
Sunday	Off		

Table 9.7 Muscle Phase Week 5: Block 2 Microcycle 1

Perform initial sets at an RPE of 8 to 9 and take the last set to the point of concentric muscle failure.

Day	Target muscles	Exercises	Page #
Monday	Upper body	Barbell chest press (4 sets @ 10-12RM)	47
		Dumbbell incline fly (3 sets @ 10-12RM)	52
		Reverse-grip lat pull-down (4 sets @ 10-12RM)	40
		Cable wide-grip seated row (3 sets @ 10-12RM)	34
		Dumbbell shoulder press (4 sets @ 10-12RM)	76
		Cable lateral raise (3 sets @ 10-12RM)	80
		Barbell drag curl (4 sets @ 10-12RM)	96
		Dumbbell overhead triceps extension (4 sets @ 10-12RM)	100
Tuesday	Lower body	Barbell split squat (4 sets @ 10-12RM)	120
		Leg extension (4 sets @ 10-12RM)	131
		Barbell stiff-legged deadlift (4 sets @ 10-12RM)	127
		Lying leg curl (4 sets @ 10-12RM)	133
		Machine standing calf raise (3 sets @ 10-12RM)	138
		Machine seated calf raise (3 sets @ 10-12RM)	137
		Barbell rollout (4 sets @ 10-12RM)	71
		Cable rope kneeling twisting crunch (3 sets @ 10-12RM)	62
Wednesday	Off		
Thursday	Upper body	Machine incline press (4 sets @ 10-12RM)	49
		Pec deck fly (3 sets @ 10-12RM)	53
		Pull-up (4 sets @ 10-12RM)	37
		T-bar row (3 sets @ 10-12RM)	28
		Arnold press (4 sets @ 10-12RM)	74
		Cable kneeling reverse fly (3 sets @ 10-12RM)	84
		Dumbbell standing biceps curl (4 sets @ 10-12RM)	87
		Dumbbell triceps kickback (4 sets @ 10-12RM)	104
Friday	Lower body	Leg press (4 sets @ 10-12RM)	122
		Dumbbell side lunge (4 sets @ 10-12RM)	116
		Hyperextension (4 sets @ 10-12RM)	129
		Machine seated leg curl (4 sets @ 10-12RM)	135
		Machine seated calf raise (3 sets @ 10-12RM)	137
		Toe press (3 sets @ 10-12RM)	136
		Cable rope kneeling crunch (4 sets @ 10-12RM)	61
		Cable wood chop (3 sets @ 10-12RM)	70
Saturday	Off		
Sunday	Off		

Table 9.8 Muscle Phase Week 6: Block 2 Microcycle 2

Perform initial sets at an RPE of 8 to 9 and take the last set to the point of concentric muscle failure.

Day	Target muscles	Exercises	Page #
Monday	Upper body	Dumbbell incline press (4 sets @ 8-10RM)	43
		Chest dip (3 sets @ 8-10RM)	55
		Cross cable lat pull-down (4 sets @ 8-10RM)	42
		Dumbbell pullover (3 sets @ 8-10RM)	26
		Cable upright row (4 sets @ 8-10RM)	86
		Dumbbell bent reverse fly (3 sets @ 8-10RM)	81
		Dumbbell standing hammer curl (4 sets @ 8-10RM)	94
		Cable rope overhead triceps extension (4 sets @ 8-10RM)	101
Tuesday	Lower body	Barbell front squat (4 sets @ 8-10RM)	118
		Sissy squat (4 sets @ 8-10RM)	125
		Good morning (4 sets @ 8-10RM)	124
		Machine kneeling leg curl (4 sets @ 8-10RM)	134
		Machine standing calf raise (3 sets @ 8-10RM)	138
		Machine seated calf raise (3 sets @ 8-10RM)	137
		Cable rope kneeling crunch (4 sets @ 8-10RM)	61
		Roman chair side crunch (3 sets @ 8-10RM)	59
Wednesday	Off		
Thursday	Upper body	Barbell decline press (4 sets @ 8-10RM)	48
		Cable fly (3 sets @ 8-10RM)	54
		Lat pull-down (4 sets @ 8-10RM)	38
		Barbell reverse-grip bent row (3 sets @ 8-10RM)	29
		Machine shoulder press (4 sets @ 8-10RM)	77
		Cable lateral raise (3 sets @ 8-10RM)	80
		Concentration curl (4 sets @ 8-10RM)	93
		Machine triceps dip (4 sets @ 8-10RM)	109
Friday	Lower body	Barbell lunge (4 sets @ 8-10RM)	113
		Dumbbell step-up (4 sets @ 8-10RM)	117
		Reverse hyperextension (4 sets @ 8-10RM)	130
		Lying leg curl (4 sets @ 8-10RM)	133
		Machine seated calf raise (3 sets @ 8-10RM)	137
		Machine standing calf raise (3 sets @ 8-10RM)	138
		Reverse crunch (4 sets @ 8-10RM)	57
		Russian twist (3 sets @ 8-10RM)	67
Saturday	Off		
Sunday	Off		

Table 9.9 Muscle Phase Week 7: Block 2 Microcycle 3

Perform all sets to the point of concentric muscle failure.

Day	Target muscles	Exercises	Page #
Monday	Upper body	Barbell incline press (4 sets @ 6-8RM)	46
		Dumbbell flat fly (3 sets @ 6-8RM)	51
		Chin-up (4 sets @ 6-8RM)	36
		Machine close-grip seated row (3 sets @ 6-8RM)	31
		Military press (4 sets @ 6-8RM)	75
		Machine lateral raise (3 sets @ 6-8RM)	79
		Cable curl (4 sets @ 6-8RM)	98
		Cable triceps press-down (4 sets @ 6-8RM)	107
Tuesday	Lower body	Bulgarian squat (4 sets @ 6-8RM)	121
		Barbell split squat (4 sets @ 6-8RM)	120
		Cable glute kickback (4 sets @ 6-8RM)	128
		Machine seated leg curl (4 sets @ 6-8RM)	135
		Toe press (3 sets @ 6-8RM)	136
		Machine seated calf raise (3 sets @ 6-8RM)	137
		Hanging knee raise (4 sets @ 6-8RM)	66
		Dumbbell side bend (3 sets @ 6-8RM)	68
Wednesday	Off		
Thursday	Upper body	Dumbbell chest press (4 sets @ 6-8RM)	45
		Pec deck fly (3 sets @ 6-8RM)	53
		Lat pull-down (4 sets @ 6-8RM)	38
		Neutral-grip lat pull-down (3 sets @ 6-8RM)	39
		Dumbbell shoulder press (4 sets @ 6-8RM)	76
		Dumbbell lateral raise (3 sets @ 6-8RM)	78
		Dumbbell incline biceps curl (4 sets @ 6-8RM)	88
		Nosebreaker (4 sets @ 6-8RM)	102
Friday	Lower body	Dumbbell reverse lunge (4 sets @ 6-8RM)	115
		One-leg extension (4 sets @ 6-8RM)	132
		Dumbbell stiff-legged deadlift (4 sets @ 6-8RM)	127
		Machine kneeling leg curl (4 sets @ 6-8RM)	134
		Machine standing calf raise (3 sets @ 6-8RM)	138
		Machine seated calf raise (3 sets @ 6-8RM)	137
		Toe touch (4 sets @ 6-8RM)	63
		Cable side bend (3 sets @ 6-8RM)	69
Saturday	Off		
Sunday	Off		

Table 9.10   Muscle Phase Week 8: Block 2 Microcycle 4

Perform these exercises at an RPE of 7.

Day	Target muscles	Exercises	Page #
Monday	Total body	Barbell chest press (3 sets @ 15-20RM)	47
		Machine close-grip seated row (3 sets @ 15-20RM)	31
		Arnold press (3 sets @ 15-20RM)	74
		Barbell preacher curl (3 sets @ 15-20RM)	91
		Dumbbell overhead triceps extension (3 sets @ 15-20RM)	100
		Barbell front squat (3 sets @ 15-20RM)	118
		Good morning (3 sets @ 15-20RM)	124
		Machine standing calf raise (3 sets @ 15-20RM)	138
		Plank (3 sets @ 30 sec static hold)	64
Tuesday	Off		
Wednesday	Off		
Thursday	Total body	Dumbbell incline fly (3 sets @ 15-20RM)	52
		Cross cable lat pull-down (3 sets @ 15-20RM)	42
		Machine shoulder press (3 sets @ 15-20RM)	77
		Cable rope hammer curl (3 sets @ 15-20RM)	97
		Cable triceps kickback (3 sets @ 15-20RM)	105
		Dumbbell lunge (3 sets @ 15-20RM)	114
		Lying leg curl (3 sets @ 15-20RM)	133
		Toe press (3 sets @ 15-20RM)	136
		Side bridge (3 sets @ 30 sec static hold)	65
Friday	Off		
Saturday	Off		
Sunday	Off		

Table 9.11 Muscle Phase Week 9: Block 3 Microcycle 1

Perform all sets to the point of concentric muscle failure.

Day	Target muscles	Exercises	Page #
Monday	Back, chest, abdomen	Lat pull-down supersetted with barbell incline press (4 sets @ 10-12RM)	38 and 46
		Dumbbell one-arm row supersetted with dumbbell decline press (4 sets @ 10-12RM)	27 and 44
		Dumbbell pullover supersetted with cable fly (3 sets @ 10-12RM)	26 and 54
		Stability ball abdominal crunch (4 sets @ 10-12RM)	60
		Russian twist (4 sets @ 10-12RM)	67
Tuesday	Legs	Barbell back squat supersetted with barbell stiff-legged deadlift (4 sets @ 10-12RM)	119 and 126
		Dumbbell side lunge supersetted with machine seated leg curl (4 sets @ 10-12RM)	116 and 135
		Sissy squat supersetted with cable glute kickback (3 sets @ 10-12RM)	125 and 128
		Machine standing calf raise (4 sets @ 10-12RM)	138
		Machine seated calf raise (3 sets @ 10-12RM)	137
Wednesday	Shoulders, arms	Military press (4 sets @ 10-12RM)	75
		Machine lateral raise (4 sets @ 10-12RM)	79
		Machine rear delt fly (4 sets @ 10-12RM)	82
		Cable rope overhead triceps extension supersetted with cable rope hammer curl (3 sets @ 10-12RM)	101 and 97
		Nosebreaker supersetted with barbell drag curl (2 sets @ 10-12RM)	102 and 96
		Dumbbell triceps kickback supersetted with dumbbell facedown incline curl (2 sets @ 10-12RM)	104 and 89
Thursday	Off		

(continued)

Table 9.11 (*continued*)

Day	Target muscles	Exercises	Page #
Friday	Back, chest, abdomen	Chin-up supersetted with dumbbell incline press (4 sets @ 10-12RM)	36 and 43
		Cable seated row supersetted with barbell chest press (4 sets @ 10-12RM)	33 and 47
		Cable straight-arm lat pull-down supersetted with pec deck fly (3 sets @ 10-12RM)	41 and 53
		Cable rope kneeling crunch (4 sets @ 10-12RM)	61
		Hanging knee raise (4 sets @ 10-12RM)	66
Saturday	Legs	Barbell front squat supersetted with hyperextension (4 sets @ 10-12RM)	118 and 129
		Dumbbell reverse lunge supersetted with reverse hyperextension (4 sets @ 10-12RM)	115 and 130
		Leg extension supersetted with machine kneeling leg curl (3 sets @ 10-12RM)	131 and 134
		Machine standing calf raise (4 sets @ 10-12RM)	138
		Machine seated calf raise (3 sets @ 10-12RM)	137
Sunday	Shoulders, arms	Dumbbell shoulder press (4 sets @ 10-12RM)	76
		Cable lateral raise (3 sets @ 10-12RM)	80
		Machine rear delt fly (3 sets @ 10-12RM)	82
		Cable triceps press-down supersetted with dumbbell incline biceps curl (3 sets @ 10-12RM)	107 and 88
		Machine nosebreaker supersetted with concentration curl (2 sets @ 10-12RM)	103 and 93
		Triceps dip supersetted with dumbbell standing hammer curl (2 sets @ 10-12RM)	108 and 94

Table 9.12 Muscle Phase Week 10: Block 3 Microcycle 2

Perform all sets to the point of concentric muscle failure.

Day	Target muscles	Exercises	Page #
Monday	Back, chest, abdomen	Cross cable lat pull-down (4 sets @ 6-8RM)	42
		Reverse-grip lat pull-down (4 sets @ 6-8RM)	40
		Machine wide-grip seated row (3 sets @ 6-8RM)	32
		Barbell chest press (4 sets @ 6-8RM)	47
		Dumbbell incline press (4 sets @ 6-8RM)	43
		Pec deck fly (3 sets @ 6-8RM)	53
		Reverse crunch (4 sets @ 6-8RM)	57
		Cable wood chop (4 sets @ 6-8RM)	70
Tuesday	Legs	Leg press (4 sets @ 6-8RM)	122
		Dumbbell lunge (4 sets @ 6-8RM)	114
		One-leg extension (3 sets @ 6-8RM)	132
		Good morning (4 sets @ 6-8RM)	124
		Lying leg curl (4 sets @ 6-8RM)	133
		Machine seated calf raise (4 sets @ 6-8RM)	137
		Machine standing calf raise (3 sets @ 6-8RM)	138
Wednesday	Shoulders, arms	Arnold press (4 sets @ 6-8RM)	74
		Dumbbell lateral raise (4 sets @ 6-8RM)	78
		Cable reverse fly (4 sets @ 6-8RM)	83
		Cable rope overhead triceps extension (4 sets @ 6-8RM)	101
		Cable triceps kickback (3 sets @ 6-8RM)	105
		Barbell preacher curl (4 sets @ 6-8RM)	91
		Dumbbell standing biceps curl (3 sets @ 6-8RM)	87
Thursday	Off		
Friday	Back, chest, abdomen	Lat pull-down—V-bar variation (4 sets @ 6-8RM)	38
		Dumbbell one-arm row (4 sets @ 6-8RM)	27
		Dumbbell pullover (3 sets @ 6-8RM)	26
		Dumbbell incline press (4 sets @ 6-8RM)	43
		Barbell decline press (4 sets @ 6-8RM)	48
		Cable fly (3 sets @ 6-8RM)	54
		Cable rope kneeling twisting crunch (4 sets @ 6-8RM)	62
		Roman chair side crunch (4 sets @ 6-8RM)	59

(continued)

Table 9.12 (*continued*)

Day	Target muscles	Exercises	Page #
Saturday	Legs	Barbell back squat (4 sets @ 6-8RM)	119
		Dumbbell step-up (4 sets @ 6-8RM)	117
		Sissy squat (4 sets @ 6-8RM)	125
		Good morning (4 sets @ 6-8RM)	124
		Lying leg curl (4 sets @ 6-8RM)	133
		Machine seated calf raise (4 sets @ 6-8RM)	137
		Machine standing calf raise (3 sets @ 6-8RM)	138
Sunday	Shoulders, arms	Military press (4 sets @ 6-8RM)	75
		Cable upright row (4 sets @ 6-8RM)	86
		Machine rear delt fly (4 sets @ 6-8RM)	82
		Cable triceps press-down (4 sets @ 6-8RM)	107
		Nosebreaker (3 sets @ 6-8RM)	102
		Cable curl (4 sets @ 6-8RM)	98
		Concentration curl (3 sets @ 6-8RM)	93

CHAPTER 10

MAX Nutrition

As you're probably aware, training and nutrition go hand in hand. Some fitness pros go as far as to say that diet is responsible for 90 percent of your body composition. Although this might be a bit of a stretch, one thing is certain: Proper nutrition is vital to maximizing muscle development. You must eat to grow!

Because it would take an entire book to detail the complexities of nutrition science as it relates to gaining muscle, this chapter covers only the basics. What follows is an overview of the primary dietary factors that affect muscle development—namely, calories and macronutrients (protein, carbohydrate, and fat). Theories about how many calories and which foods to consume in which quantities abound. Many are based on myth and misinterpretation. The information presented here will help you determine what to eat and in what quantities and explain how and why your nutritional choices make a difference.

From a muscle-development standpoint, when you eat is arguably as important as what you eat. This concept, called *nutrient timing*, has been extensively investigated by researchers, and studies consistently show that consuming nutrients during and around your training session has a greater effect on anabolism than consuming them at other times of the day. Do not take this to mean that general nutrition principles are unimportant from a hypertrophy standpoint. Quite the contrary. Still, you must consider timing in order to optimize muscle growth. Later in this chapter I provide guidelines for what to eat before, during, and after your workouts.

NUTRITIONAL RECOMMENDATIONS

Consider the following recommendations as flexible guidelines for creating a customized muscle-building diet rather than unyielding nutrition principles. Although these recommendations are grounded in science, take into account your own preferences, goals, and experiences. There is a great deal of variance in how people respond to different foods. Some trial and error are required to determine your optimal caloric intake and macronutrient ratios. Be prepared to experiment until you get it right.

Calories

As a general rule, you need to consume a surplus of calories in order to build muscle. This is consistent with the first law of thermodynamics, which states that energy can be neither created nor destroyed, only changed from one form to another. In simpler terms, the first law of thermodynamics can be expressed by the following equation:

$$\text{calories in} - \text{calories out} = \text{change in body mass}.$$

The ramifications of this equation are clear: When you take in more calories than you expend, the excess energy is stored in the form of body mass. Whether the additional mass is muscle or fat depends on a host of diet- and training-related factors.

Old-school mass-gaining regimens consisted of alternating cycles of bulking and cutting. During the bulking cycles, lifters would scarf down everything imaginable, paying little heed to the types of foods consumed. Triple cheeseburgers, fries, ice cream, cookies ... the more calorically rich the food, the better. This unfettered gluttony was then followed by a period of extreme dieting in which the lifters would cut calories to a bare minimum in an effort to lean out. In a perfect world, the strategy would end up leaving you huge and shredded.

Unfortunately, we don't live in a perfect world. Sure, the bulking and cutting approach significantly helps to increase body mass. I've known a few pro bodybuilders who put on upward of 100 pounds (45 kg) in the bulking phase. There's one little problem with these results, though: as much as 75 percent of the weight is in the form of body fat. Unless you plan to compete as a sumo wrestler, that's far too much. It can take up to a year or more to diet down to an acceptable level of body fat. Worse, hard-earned muscle is inevitably sacrificed in the dieting process. You're lucky to hold on to half of your muscle gains. It's a poor cost–benefit ratio.

Of even greater concern is that the bulking and cutting approach is detrimental to long-term body composition. This appears to be a function of your biological set point. Simply stated, set point is the body's way of physiologically regulating your weight. Through various processes, your body makes a coordinated effort to adjust the intake and expenditure of energy so that a specified amount of fat stores are maintained. Any attempt to deviate from this predetermined level is actively resisted. As you may imagine, chronic dieting is perceived as a threat to your energy reserves. Accordingly, your body continually trains itself to survive on fewer and fewer calories during each cycle of yo-yo dieting. In an attempt to maintain homeostasis, it alters various hormonal and enzymatic mechanisms; in certain cases, these alterations can be difficult to reverse. Inevitably, your biological set point goes up, resulting in a predisposition to retain higher levels of body fat in future cycles.

The key to a successful muscle-building diet is to keep calories in a range that promotes the development of lean mass rather than body fat. A gain of about 1 pound (0.5 kg) of muscle per week is the upper limit of what you can expect to attain without fattening up in the process. For those who have several years of training experience, a gain of about 0.5 pound (0.25 kg) of muscle per week is probably more realistic.

How many calories should you consume to achieve lean gains? A good estimate is to take in 18 to 20 calories per pound (40 per kg) of body weight. For example, if you weigh 200 pounds (91 kg), your target caloric intake is approximately 3,600 to 4,000 calories per day. Understand that this is a general guideline. Those who easily gain fat typically do better with a slightly lower caloric intake, whereas hard gainers who have difficulty packing on muscle may need to consume significantly more—perhaps as much 25 calories per pound of body weight. You'll need to experiment with different caloric intakes to find out what works best for you.

It's essential to approach this process in a systematic manner. I like to use the rule of 100. Start off by consuming 18 to 20 calories per pound of body weight for a month or so. If you aren't gaining enough mass, increase your intake by an additional 100 calories per day. If, on the other hand, you are gaining too much fat, cut back your intake by 100 calories per day. Evaluate your progress after a few weeks and continue tweaking in 100-calorie increments as needed. Making these adjustments in a controlled fashion will allow you to fine tune your diet so that you can optimize the ratio of muscle gains to fat gains.

Protein

From a muscle-building perspective, protein can be considered the king of all nutrients. The amino acids in dietary protein sources are the building blocks of muscle tissue, and their presence is required for anabolic signaling pathways to carry out protein synthesis.

Amino acids are divided into two basic categories: essential and nonessential. The essential amino acids (leucine, tryptophan, lysine, methionine, phenylalanine, threonine, valine, histidine, and isoleucine) are the most nutritionally significant. The body cannot manufacture these amino acids; therefore, you must obtain them from the foods in your diet. A dietary shortage in even one of the essential amino acids is enough to impair your muscle development.

Protein status in the body is determined by nitrogen balance. A negative nitrogen balance means that your body is breaking down proteins at a greater rate than it's synthesizing them; a positive nitrogen balance means that your body is creating new proteins faster than it is breaking them down; and a stable nitrogen balance means that protein degradation and protein synthesis are in equilibrium.

To build muscle, you need to be in a positive nitrogen balance. This requires adhering to a protein-rich diet. If your intake of protein is insufficient to make up for what you excrete, cellular function is compromised and muscle development suffers. Only by consuming protein in excess of losses can you promote anabolism and enhance lean muscle development.

The recommended dietary allowance (RDA) for protein is equal to a little less than 0.4 gram of protein per pound of body weight. Not a heck of a lot. One little caveat: The RDA bases protein requirements on the needs of the average couch potato. Although this is fine if you want to be an average couch potato, it has little relevance if your goal is to maximize muscle development.

Studies on nitrogen balance indicate that people involved in serious resistance training programs require a protein intake of about 0.7 to 0.9 grams per pound (1.6 to 2.0 grams/kg) of body weight (Campbell et al. 2007). Although this probably suffices for most lifters, my general recommendation is to round these numbers up and consume approximately 1 gram of protein per pound of body weight. For example, if you weigh 200 pounds (91 kg), protein intake should equal approximately 200 grams per day. This provides a margin of safety, ensuring that you never fall into negative nitrogen balance. There really is no downside to the approach. Taking in a little extra protein won't hurt; not getting enough surely will.

I've heard some fitness pros claim that a significantly greater protein intake—as much as 2 grams per pound of body weight—is required to maximize muscle gains. This recommendation may have credence for those who take performance-enhancing drugs; however, it is excessive if you're not chemically enhanced. The body has a limited capacity to utilize protein for tissue-building purposes, and there's no way to store it for future use. Once this saturation point is reached, additional protein is of no use to your muscles and is either burned off as energy or converted into glucose or fat.

Much has been made about the importance of consuming high-quality proteins for building muscle. Supplement companies, in particular, have perpetuated the belief that protein quality is paramount, citing qualitative measurement scales such as biological value and protein efficiency ratio to bolster their case. The claims make for good ad copy, but generally speaking they're wildly overstated.

The quality of a protein is largely a function of its composition of essential amino acids, both in terms of quantity and proportion. A complete protein contains a full complement of all nine essential amino acids in the approximate amounts needed by the body. Conversely, proteins that are low in one or more of the essential amino acids are considered incomplete.

With the exception of gelatin, all animal-based proteins (meats, dairy products, eggs, and so on) are complete proteins. Assuming that you eat a variety of animal-based foods (and follow my recommendation for consuming one gram of protein per pound of body weight), qualitative issues are basically moot; you are assured of getting all the essential amino acids you need for optimal development. The one time during which the type of protein consumed is potentially important is during and around a workout. I discuss this later in this chapter.

Vegetable-based proteins, on the other hand, lack various essential amino acids; therefore, they are incomplete. This isn't really an issue for lacto-ovo vegetarians because eggs and dairy products are excellent protein sources and have a full complement of amino acids. Vegans, on the other hand, have to be a little more watchful. They need to eat the right combination of foods to ensure that they obtain adequate essential amino acids through the diet. For instance, grains are limited in lysine and threonine whereas legumes are low in methionine. Combining the two offsets the weakness of each and thereby helps prevent a deficiency. Note that these foods don't necessarily have to be eaten in the same meal; they just need to be included in the diet on a regular basis.

Carbohydrate

The recent low-carbohydrate craze has perpetuated a belief that carbohydrate is responsible for pretty much every dietary-related health issue known to humans. This premise has spawned an entire industry of best-selling books and low-carbohydrate supplements that promote the anti-carbohydrate sentiment. As a result, carbophobia runs rampant in a large segment of the population. This is especially true of bodybuilders and other physique athletes, who often hold fast to the belief that reducing carbohydrate intake is the key to staying lean.

Let's be clear: Losing body fat is far more complex than simply eliminating carbohydrate from your diet. Carbohydrate, when eaten sensibly, can and should be an integral part of your dietary regimen. This is particularly true when your goal is to build muscle. To understand why, it's necessary to delve into a little nutritional physiology.

The compounds derived from carbohydrate breakdown are stored as glycogen in your muscles and liver. Glycogen is the primary fuel used to power your muscles during resistance training workouts. It provides an instant source of energy that can be accessed on demand, enabling you to work out at an intense level. When glycogen stores are depleted (as happens when you follow a diet very low in carbohydrate), your body coverts amino acids into glucose in order to meet short-term energy needs. However, this conversion process is very inefficient and fails to supply adequate fuel for training. Within a short period of time, your stamina begins to wane and you lose the ability to train at peak efficiency.

Worse, studies show that training in a glycogen-depleted state has a catabolic effect on muscle (Churchley et al. 2007). Low glycogen levels alter cellular signaling pathways, impairing protein synthesis and reducing the effectiveness of the genes responsible for regulating muscle growth. The take-away message is that you simply won't maximize muscle development without including a healthy amount of carbohydrate in your diet.

For muscle-building purposes, most people seem to do best consuming 2 to 3 grams of carbohydrate per pound of body weight. Because each gram of carbohydrate contains 4 calories, this translates to a daily carbohydrate intake of approximately 1,600 to 2,400 calories. Those who are insulin insensitive (characterized by an impaired ability to store carbohydrate in the muscles) may require a somewhat lower intake to avoid excess fat storage—perhaps as low as 1 gram per pound of body weight per day. Experiment with different amounts and see what works best for you.

All types of carbohydrate, however, are not created equal. Some are better than others for maximizing muscle development while minimizing fat deposition. The best way to determine which types to eat and which to avoid is to assess their nutrient density, which takes into account the amount of vitamins and minerals as well as fiber in a food source. Nutrient-dense carbohydrate foods are insulin friendly and they supply your body with essential compounds that enhance metabolic function. Many of the vitamins and minerals in these foods are used as cofactors that assist the body in burning fat. Others are antioxidants that keep cells functioning optimally. Fiber promotes satiety, decreasing the urge to pig out on junk food.

In contrast, carbohydrate foods that are not nutrient dense are basically empty calories. The worst offenders are processed foods containing carbohydrate. They contribute virtually nothing to biological function and send blood sugar levels sky high. Making matters worse, excessive consumption of these foods can exacerbate insulin resistance. When large amounts of insulin are stimulated on a repeated basis, glucose receptors are forced to work overtime. Eventually, receptors become desensitized to insulin and glucose cannot be stored as efficiently. The net result is an increased propensity to store fat.

Which types of carbohydrate can be considered nutrient dense? Fruits and vegetables are at the top of the list. In addition to being rich in vitamins, minerals, and fiber, they contain substances called phytochemicals. These compounds, which go by obscure names such as indoles and isothiocyanates, are rapidly becoming one of the most exciting areas in the field of nutrition. Research is still emerging, but phytochemicals have already been shown to provide numerous health-related benefits and are believed to have anti-aging properties. Some evidence suggests that they may play a role in muscle protein synthesis and repair (Gorelick-Feldman et al. 2008). As scientists conduct further studies, phytochemicals may very well turn out to be the closest thing yet to a nutritional fountain of youth.

Whole grains are also nutrient-dense carbohydrate foods that should be staples of a muscle-building diet. To help distinguish between whole grains and their processed counterparts, remember the slogan, "Think brown!" For example, instead of white pasta, white rice, sweetened cereals, and white-flour breads, choose whole-wheat pasta, brown rice, oatmeal, and multigrain bread. As a general rule, brown starches are not processed and thus maintain their nutrient density. They digest slowly, allowing glucose to enter the bloodstream in a time-released fashion. Ultimately, insulin remains stable, and the potential for excess fat storage is diminished.

Fat

Just as some consider carbohydrate the root of all nutritional evil, others claim that dietary fat is the biggest culprit in obesity and disease. The low-fat philosophy is predicated on the fact that dietary fat is calorically dense: each gram contains nine calories. Do the math and you'll see that you have to eat more than twice the amount of protein or carbohydrate (which both have only four calories per gram) to get the same number of calories as a given portion of fat. What's more, excess fat calories have a conversion efficiency of around 98 percent, whereas the conversion efficiency for carbohydrate is only about 70 percent, meaning that it's much easier to convert dietary fat into flab than to convert carbohydrate into flab. These factors seem to suggest that a low-fat approach is the way to go.

Unfortunately, these numbers don't tell the whole story. Fats are essential nutrients that play a vital role in many bodily functions. They are involved in cushioning your internal organs for protection, aiding in the absorption of vitamins, and facilitating the production of cell membranes, hormones, and prostaglandins. Depending on the extent of restriction, low-fat diets can fail to supply the necessary nutrients to keep your body running at peak efficiency.

Low-fat diets are particularly detrimental to building muscle. Fat consumption is positively associated with testosterone production; if fat intake is restricted, testosterone levels decline. Studies show that the correlation between testosterone levels and fat intake is especially strong in experienced lifters (Sallinen et al. 2004). The implication is clear: Follow a low-fat diet and you impair muscle growth.

Taking all factors into account, a moderate approach to fat consumption is warranted. A good rule of thumb is to consume at least 20 percent of calories from fat. Given that mass-building diets require a surplus of calories, this should be easy to accomplish.

Because protein intake is always a constant (approximately 1 gram per pound of body weight), the actual number of fat grams consumed is inversely correlated with carbohydrate intake: Consume more carbohydrate and you'll consume less dietary fat, and vice versa. To determine actual intake, figure out your protein and carbohydrate consumption; your fat consumption will be whatever is left over. Say, for example, that you weigh 200 pounds (91 kg) and your target is 4,000 calories per day. If you consume 2 grams of carbohydrate per pound of body weight at 4 calories per gram (1,600 calories) and 1 gram of protein per pound of body weight at 4 calories per gram (800 calories), then daily fat intake would equal 1,600 calories. Because fat has 9 calories per gram, this would equal approximately 178 grams of fat. If you increase carbohydrate intake to 3 grams per pound of body weight, then you reduce fat intake to 800 calories (approximately 89 grams of fat).

The majority of your fats should come from unsaturated sources. Unsaturated fats help maintain fluidity in cell membranes, allowing hormones and other chemical messengers to readily penetrate the cells. This has wide-ranging effects, from increasing muscle protein synthesis to improving insulin sensitivity to enhancing fat utilization.

Monounsaturated fats (found in olive oil and various nuts) and the long-chain omega-3 fats derived from fatty fish are particularly beneficial to cellular processes. In addition to their role in anabolic function, these fats possess health-related benefits that span virtually every organ system in your body. Suffice to say, they should make up the majority of your dietary fat intake.

There is conflicting evidence about the effects of the intake of saturated fat—found primarily in meats and dairy—on markers of health. Some studies show a strong link to cardiovascular diseases and certain types of cancers whereas others do not. A complete discussion of the topic is beyond the scope of this book.

Regardless of health implications, saturated fats contribute little to bodily processes. If not used immediately for energy, they're shuttled with a high degree of efficiency into fat cells for long-term storage. Numerous studies have demonstrated that given the same caloric intake, eating saturated fats results in a greater body fat deposition than eating unsaturated fats. Moreover, evidence shows that a high intake of saturated fat can reduce insulin sensitivity (Rivellese, De Natale, and Lilli 2002). Bottom line: Focus on consuming unsaturated fats and keep saturated fat intake to a minimum.

Summary of MAX Nutritional Recommendations

- Consume approximately 18 to 20 calories per pound of body weight. Those who store fat easily may need slightly fewer calories, whereas hard gainers will likely need substantially more.
- Consume approximately one gram of protein per pound of body weight.
- Consume approximately two to three grams of carbohydrate per pound of body weight. The majority should come from nutrient-dense sources, including whole grains, fruits, and vegetables.
- After you determine carbohydrate and protein intake, fat intake will constitute the remaining calories in your diet. A minimum intake of approximately 20 percent of total calories is recommended. The majority of fats should come from unsaturated sources, particularly monounsaturated fats and omega-3 fats.

NUTRIENT TIMING

Now that you have a handle on the foods to eat to build muscle, let's delve into the all-important topic of optimizing the timing of nutrient consumption. Here's a rundown of preworkout, during-workout, and postworkout nutritional guidelines that support your muscle-building efforts. As noted previously, people are unique in their responses to various food sources. Thus, a little experimentation may be necessary to optimize both the types and quantity of food you consume before, during, and after your workouts.

What to Eat Before a Workout

The main nutritional goal preworkout is to supply adequate energy for your muscles and brain during training. This makes carbohydrate consumption essential. Because intense exercise utilizes energy at a very fast rate, the body can't supply enough oxygen to harness fat as a fuel source. It therefore relies on glycogen (stored carbohydrate), which doesn't require oxygen to be broken down for energy.

By taking in an ample amount of carbohydrate before exercise, you ensure that your body's glycogen stores are fully stocked. It's estimated that more than 80 percent of energy in a bodybuilding-style workout is obtained from the breakdown of glycogen. Only by maintaining a ready supply of glycogen can you train in an all-out fashion and extend performance without hitting the wall.

If that's not enough of a reason to consume carbohydrate before a workout, consider this: Training in a glycogen-depleted state blunts anabolism. Multiple studies show that protein synthesis slows to a crawl when glycogen stores are low (Churchley et al. 2007; Creer et al. 2005). This is likely a survival mechanism. Without sufficient glycogen to fuel activity, your body tries to spare energy by blocking anabolic signaling pathways. Making matters worse, cortisol, a catabolic stress hormone, is secreted in an attempt to mobilize additional fuel. Suffice to say, you're not going to build much muscle in this scenario.

You should also include protein in your preworkout meal. Consuming protein before exercise has both anabolic and anticatabolic effects. By providing a steady stream of amino acids at the onset of training, you maximize their delivery to working muscles and thereby attenuate the breakdown of muscle tissue during your workout. Some evidence even shows that consuming protein before exercise significantly increases muscle protein synthesis in the first hour *after* exercise, priming the body for anabolism. The validity of this claim needs further study.

Fat, on the other hand, is not nutritionally significant in the preworkout period. In fact, you may want to limit its consumption. Fat delays gastric emptying, thereby prolonging the time it takes food to digest. If food sits in your stomach during exercise, you face an increased likelihood of gastric problems, including cramping, nausea, and reflux. If you consume the pre-workout meal at least a couple of hours or more before training, however, this should not be much of an issue.

Ideally, your preworkout meal should contain a nutrient-dense starch and a low-fat protein source. Turkey on multigrain bread, lean steak and yams, eggs and oatmeal, and chicken and brown rice are all good options. Total calories should be about the same as in one of your regular meals. This will provide adequate fuel without bogging down your stomach.

Try to consume your preworkout meal approximately two to three hours before training. Allowing a couple hours between the end of your meal and the onset of exercise will ensure that the majority of your meal is digested and help prevent gastric upset.

Consider eating a large piece of fruit within half an hour of training. Fruits are generally low on the glycemic index scale, meaning that they don't cause a rapid spike in blood sugar. This is significant because insulin levels stay stable, thereby preventing the potential for rebound hypoglycemia—a condition that can result in lightheadedness and fatigue. At the same time, fruits provide a valuable source of fuel during exercise, improving your capacity to train. Apples, pears, strawberries, and other low-glycemic fruits make excellent choices.

Ideally, you should combine the piece of fruit with a whey protein drink. Whey is a fast-acting protein, meaning that it's rapidly absorbed into circulation. This expedites the flow of amino acids to your muscles without having an appreciable effect on digestion. Aim for about 0.1 gram of whey, mixed in a water-based solution, per pound of body weight. A person who weighs 150 pounds (68 kg) would need about 15 grams of whey. You can combine the fruit with the whey in a shake for easy digestion.

This also is a great time to have a nice big cup or two of coffee. Caffeine stimulates the central nervous system, increasing your ability to produce muscular force. Caffeine also blocks pain receptors in the brain, allowing you to train harder for longer. These performance-enhancing effects can provide that extra edge to help you take your workout to the next level.

What to Eat During a Workout

The most important nutrient to consume during MAX training is water. As you work out, you lose water through your sweat, breath, and perhaps urine. If you don't replenish these fluids, your exercise performance is bound to suffer. In fact, decrements in muscle strength can manifest after only a 2 percent reduction in hydration status. This is especially problematic if you're training in a hot environment.

It is a mistake, however, to rely on thirst as an indicator of when to drink. Intense exercise inhibits the thirst sensors in your throat and gut; by the time you become thirsty, your body is already dehydrated. This is compounded by the fact that your thirst sensors become less and less sensitive as you age.

The general rule during exercise is to drink early and drink often. Consume 8 ounces of fluid immediately before your workout and then take small sips of water every 15 or 20 minutes while training, varying the volume based on sweating rate. This will ensure a continued state of hydration, keeping fluid balance intact.

What to Eat After a Workout

The postexercise meal is perhaps the most important meal of all. After an intense workout, your body is in a catabolic state. It has spent a good deal of its stored fuels (including glycogen and amino acids) and sustained damage to its muscle fibers. The good news is that this presents a window of opportunity for anabolism. By consuming the proper ratio of nutrients during this time, not only do you initiate the rebuilding of damaged tissue and energy reserves, you do so in a supercompensated fashion that fosters improvements in both body composition and exercise performance.

One of the primary goals after exercise is to replenish glycogen stores. Because glucose is depleted during training, your muscles and liver are literally starved for carbohydrate. In response, several adaptations take place. Glucose transporters (specifically GLUT-4) responsible for bringing glucose into muscle cells become much more active, and your body stimulates the activity of glycogen synthase—the principal enzyme involved in promoting glycogen storage. The combination of these factors facilitates the rapid uptake of glucose, allowing glycogen to be replenished at an accelerated rate.

Carbohydrate is best taken in liquid form and should come from simple, high-glycemic sources. This is one instance in which it is beneficial to spike insulin levels. You see, insulin has both anabolic and anticatabolic functions, helping to increase protein synthesis, decrease protein breakdown, and shuttle glycogen into cells. And this is one instance in which increased insulin won't promote increases in body fat. Because your muscles are in a depleted state, nutrients tend to be used for purposes of lean tissue rather than fat storage.

A combination of glucose and fructose is ideal. In addition to potentiating an insulin response, glucose is the primary source of muscle glycogen. Fructose, on the other hand, preferentially replenishes liver glycogen. (Glucose is of limited utility to the liver, a phenomenon called the glucose paradox.) Thus, the two types of sugar work synergistically to restock the body's glycogen stores.

Grape and cranberry juices generally are good choices because they have a high ratio of glucose to fructose. A good starting point is to consume 0.5 gram of carbohydrate per pound of ideal body weight. For example, if your goal weight is 200 pounds (91 kg), you'd consume 100 grams of carbohydrate. If you tend to be insulin insensitive, cut this amount back to 0.25 gram of carbohydrate per pound of body weight. Over time, assess how your body responds and modify the amount based on your response.

The other main nutritional objective postworkout is to supply sufficient protein for tissue repair. If protein intake is inadequate following training, recuperation is shortchanged and results are compromised. You should consume protein preferably in the form of a high-quality protein powder. The idea is to bathe your muscles in amino acids, providing them with the raw materials to facilitate recovery. The upshot is significant: When you consume amino acids after training, protein synthesis increases more than threefold over fasting conditions. In this way, you build muscle fibers back up so that they're stronger than before.

A fast-acting protein such as whey works best. Because it is rapidly assimilated, whey reaches your muscles quickly, thereby expediting repair. And because your muscles are primed for anabolism, virtually all of the protein will be utilized for rebuilding. Aim for 0.25 gram of protein per pound of body weight and mix the powder directly into your postworkout drink.

Ideally, you should consume your postworkout meal as soon as possible after training. The quicker you feed your body, the more it sops up nutrients and utilizes them for repair. Because blood flow is increased from the exercise bout, the delivery of protein and carbohydrate is enhanced, resulting in greater muscle protein synthesis.

Even if you are unable to consume your postworkout meal immediately after training, all is not lost. The window of opportunity lasts for at least a couple of hours after exercise (albeit in a somewhat diminished state), so just make sure you take in the specified nutrients as soon as you can. Don't allow this opportunity to slip away!

Summary of Nutrient Timing Protocol

- Consume a meal containing a low-glycemic carbohydrate and lean protein source about two to three hours before training. Keep fat consumption to a minimum.
- Have a large piece of fruit and some whey protein (amounting to 0.1 gram per pound of body weight) within half an hour of training.
- Consume a large cup of coffee before training.
- Consume 8 ounces of fluid immediately before your workout and then take small sips of water every 15 or 20 minutes while training.
- After training, consume a drink containing high-glycemic carbohydrate (such as grape juice or cranberry juice) and a quality protein powder. Generally, you should consume about 0.5 gram of carbohydrate per pound of body weight (0.25 gram per pound of body weight for those with decreased insulin sensitivity) and 0.25 gram of protein per pound of body weight.

CHAPTER 11

The Cardio Connection

You've learned how the MAX Muscle Plan's carefully structured combination of periodized resistance training and proper nutrition helps maximize muscle development. If you follow the program as directed, you will see terrific results.

But what about cardio or, more precisely, exercise that stresses the cardio-respiratory system? Can adding some aerobic exercise to the mix further improve results by limiting or even reducing fat deposition?

Before we tackle this question, let's first set the record straight: Resistance training alone helps keep you lean—perhaps as much or even more so than cardio. A recent study illustrates just how effective lifting weights can be as a fat-loss aid (Heden et al. 2011). The study found that subjects who performed a traditional multiset resistance training protocol expended more than 200 calories during the course of the exercise bout. Not bad, but not Earth-shattering either. The kicker, however, is that metabolism remained increased for 72 hours postworkout, resulting in an extra 300 calories burned!

The additional caloric expenditure after a workout is attributable to a phenomenon known as excess postexercise oxygen consumption (EPOC), also called the afterburn. Simply stated, EPOC is a measure of the energy your body expends to return to its homeostatic state after completing a workout. The body's processes of repairing damaged tissue, replenishing glycogen stores, clearing lactic acid, re-oxygenating blood, restoring hormonal levels, and reestablishing normal core temperature all contribute to the afterburn. Because of a high degree of metabolic stress and muscle damage, resistance training affects fat loss far beyond the workout itself—and affects fat loss to a greater extent than does cardiovascular exercise.

It gets better. Resistance training also helps keep your metabolism stoked around the clock. Muscle is metabolically active tissue. This means that your body has to work harder to maintain muscle than to maintain nonlean tissue. The exact number of calories burned for 1 pound (0.45 kg) of muscle is a subject of ongoing debate, but the figure seems to be around 30 calories per pound. Although on the surface this may not seem like that much, consider that adding just 5 pounds (2.3 kg) of lean tissue would result in losing a pound of fat every month—without changing anything whatsoever about your diet or lifestyle. A 10-pound (4.5 kg) muscle gain would effectively double the metabolic effect. Bottom line: Resistance training by itself helps keep body fat levels in check while you add lean muscle to your frame.

This doesn't mean that cardio is superfluous in the control of body weight. On the contrary, regular aerobic exercise enhances fat loss. Remember that the weight loss equation has two sides: energy intake and energy expenditure. Cardio helps increase expenditure, thus creating a negative caloric balance and shifting the body into fat-burning mode.

Interestingly, fat loss from cardio exercise seems to come from the mid-section, irrespective of dietary factors. Tightly controlled studies on rodents show that performing regular aerobic exercise significantly reduces abdominal fat even when food intake is kept constant (Laye et al. 2007). Studies on humans seem to support this finding (Kwon et al. 2010). So, if that little extra paunch just doesn't seem to go away, performing some cardio may be the ticket to help you slim down.

PROS AND CONS OF CARDIO

If you recall, the principle of specificity states that adaptations are specific to the type of training you perform. With respect to cardio, several associated adaptations can have a beneficial effect on body composition. For one, cardio helps expand your network of capillaries—the tiny blood vessels that allow nutrients to be exchanged between body tissues. Before body fat can be metabolized, it must first enter the bloodstream and then be transported to the active tissues for use as fuel. Unfortunately, blood flow tends to be poor in fatty areas, which inhibits your body's ability to harness fat from these regions. The more capillaries you have, the more efficient your body becomes in liberating and using fat, particularly from stubborn areas.

Moreover, consistent aerobic exercise expands the size and number of your mitochondria (cellular furnaces where fat burning takes place) and increases the quantity of your aerobic enzymes (bodily proteins that accelerate the fat-burning process). It also has a sensitizing effect on insulin function, facilitating a greater capacity to store carbohydrate as glycogen rather than as fat. Over time, these factors ratchet up your body's ability to burn fat.

In addition to the aforementioned fat-burning benefits, cardio helps improve recuperation from heavy training. Nutrient delivery facilitates muscle repair. How does the body deliver nutrients to tissue? Through the bloodstream! The increase in capillaries associated with aerobic exercise enhances nutrient exchange and helps nourish your muscles with the substances necessary for growth.

Further, cardio serves as a form of active recovery. During aerobic training, blood is shunted to the working muscles. This further enhances nutrient delivery and hastens the removal of metabolic waste. It's why muscle soreness tends to dissipate after performing a bout of light cardio.

The catch is that adaptations are muscle specific. If you perform only lower-body cardio, you will see the majority of benefits in your legs. To realize results in the upper body you need to perform upper-body cardio exercises. This generally shouldn't be an issue. Many cardio machines, such as elliptical trainers and Arc Trainers, now include upper-body components so that all the muscles are engaged during a workout. Simply pumping your arms while walking achieves similarly beneficial results.

With all these benefits, it seems that adding a cardio component to the MAX Muscle Plan would be a no-brainer, right? Unfortunately it's not that simple. Concurrently performing aerobic exercise and resistance training can compromise muscle growth. This has been dubbed the concurrent training effect. Depending on the specific training regimen, the negative effect on muscle development can be significant.

The problem with concurrent training is that adaptations associated with resistance training aren't necessarily compatible with those of aerobic exercise. Each type of training regimen activates and suppresses specific genes and signaling pathways, and these pathways tend to interfere with one another. The net result is an impaired adaptive response, particularly from a muscle hypertrophy standpoint. Cardio seems to impair resistance training adaptations more than vice versa.

The main culprit here is an enzyme called adenosine monophosphate kinase (AMPK). AMPK is associated with an energy-conserving pathway that regulates adenosine triphosphate (ATP), the high-energy compound that fuels all human work. When energy levels become depleted during aerobic exercise, AMPK turns on enzymes involved in carbohydrate and fatty acid metabolism to restore ATP levels. Among other things, this increases the use of fat as a fuel source. That's the good news.

The bad news is that AMPK activation also blocks an anabolic pathway called mammalian target of rapamycin (mTOR), which is critical for carrying out muscle protein synthesis. This makes biological sense because the body uses a lot of energy to make muscle proteins. This is why muscle is metabolically active tissue—a lot of ATP is consumed to maintain muscle mass. Nevertheless, the result is that muscle development suffers.

Another potential downside to concurrent training is the overtraining factor. Remember that everyone has an upper limit to how much exercise they can tolerate before overtraining sets in. Performing cardio adds to the total amount of exercise-related stress placed on your body. These stresses can overwhelm your capacity to recover and lead to an overtrained state. Overtraining is associated with heightened fatigue, reduced testosterone levels, increased cortisol (a catabolic stress hormone), and an impaired immune response. To say the least, these factors are not conducive to muscle gains.

Given this background information, let's revisit the million dollar question: Is it wise to perform cardio in conjunction with the MAX Muscle Plan? The not-so-simple answer is, it depends.

One can make a case that simply controlling caloric intake is a more sensible approach to minimizing fat deposition. I've worked with many high-level physique athletes (myself included) who performed little or no cardio and achieved high levels of muscularity while maintaining very low levels of body fat. A proper diet and regimented resistance training is often sufficient for producing desired results. Better yet, it reduces the amount of time you spend in the gym, thus affording you more time for leisure.

On the other hand, you may not want to adhere to a strict diet. Or perhaps you're genetically predisposed to holding onto stubborn fat. If so, then a properly structured concurrent training regimen can help you control weight without negatively affecting muscle gains. In fact, the improved recovery associated with cardio might slightly benefit muscle development.

To sum things up, cardio has distinct benefits and detriments that you must take into account when your goal is building muscle. Weigh the pros and cons and make an informed decision based on your individual needs and genetics.

MAX CARDIO PROTOCOL

Assuming that you decide to include a cardio component, the MAX cardio routine complements the resistance training element of the MAX Muscle Plan. Before discussing the specific cardio protocol, however, let's cover the basics. Cardio has three distinct variables: intensity, duration, and frequency.

1. **Intensity** refers to how hard you train. You can estimate aerobic training intensity in several ways. The most popular method involves taking a percentage of maximal heart rate (MHR), which is calculated by subtracting your age from 220. For example, if you are 30 years old your maximal heart rate is 190 (220 – 30 = 190). To determine training intensity, simply multiply this number by a given percentage to target training intensity. Although the heart rate method is certainly viable, I generally prefer using RPE to gauge aerobic intensity. As you already know, RPE is a measure of how hard you feel you are exercising. With respect to cardio, RPE takes into account the physical sensations you experience during exercise, including increases in heart rate, breathing rate, sweating, and muscle fatigue. Table 11.1 provides a framework for estimating your RPE when performing cardio. You'll notice that it's similar to the RPE scale we use for resistance training but that the way intensity is categorized is slightly different. Whether you choose to measure intensity by the heart rate or RPE method is completely up to you; either is fine for the purposes of the MAX Muscle Plan.

2. **Duration** refers to how long you train. As a general rule, duration is inversely related to intensity; you can go longer if you don't train as hard.

3. **Frequency** refers to how often you train. Frequency is generally expressed in terms of number of weekly aerobic sessions (although technically you could perform multiple sessions in the same day).

Table 11.1 10-Point Cardio RPE Scale

RPE	Intensity
1	No exertion at all
2	Extremely light
3	Very light
4	Somewhat light
5	Light
6	Somewhat hard
7	Hard
8	Very hard
9	Extremely hard
10	Maximal exertion

The key to ensuring that muscle is not sacrificed in a concurrent training regimen is to keep cardio intensity, duration, and frequency in moderation. This limits activation of AMPK during training and reduces the potential for overtraining.

What constitutes moderation? This depends on such factors as your individual recovery ability, the type and duration of the aerobic training, and your training experience. Accordingly, the MAX cardio protocol takes a conservative approach, erring on the side of muscle preservation rather than maximizing fat loss. Here are the particulars: Perform 30 to 45 minutes of low- to moderate-intensity, steady-state cardio (equal to approximately 60-70 percent MHR or 5-6 on the cardio RPE scale) 3 to 4 days per week. Table 11.2 summarizes the protocol.

Table 11.2 Summary of MAX Cardio Protocol

Training variable	Protocol
Intensity	60-70% MHR or 6-7 RPE
Duration	30-45 min
Frequency	3-4 days per week

High-Intensity Interval Training

I'm a big advocate of high-intensity interval training (HIIT) as a fat-loss strategy. In its simplest form, HIIT entails alternating between high-intensity and low-intensity bouts of cardio. During high-intensity intervals, you generally train at a level that exceeds your lactate threshold—the point at which lactic acid begins to accumulate in your muscles. You perform low-intensity intervals at a leisurely pace, allowing your body a chance to clear lactic acid and replenish energy.

An emerging body of research suggests that HIIT can be more effective and efficient than steady-state cardio for reducing fat (Trapp et al. 2008). On a basic level, HIIT burns more calories in less time during a workout session. If you're like me and would rather get cardio over with as soon as possible, this is a big plus. But the real fat-burning benefits come during the postexercise period. You see, EPOC is intensity dependent—the harder you train, the more calories you expend after training. With HIIT, the net effect can last for 36 hours or more postworkout, burning as many as 150 calories a day beyond resting levels.

If HIIT is the better fat burner, why do I advocate a low-intensity, steady-state cardio protocol for the MAX Muscle Plan? Because HIIT can hinder muscle development. For one, HIIT saps energy and has particularly taxing effects on the central nervous system. The highly demanding nature of interval training can make it difficult to hit the weights with an adequate intensity of effort. If your goal is to build muscle, lifting intensity is not something you want to compromise.

Moreover, combining HIIT with resistance training increases the potential for overtraining. The MAX Muscle Plan pushes your muscles to their limits on a regular basis, keeping you on the edge of overreaching. Performing cardio at high levels of intensity as you must do in an HIIT routine can send you over the edge. If you continue to perform cardio workouts at these levels for a sustained period of time, the inevitable result is an overtrained state in which muscle gains grind to a halt.

If you are seeking to optimize fat loss and don't mind sacrificing some muscle growth, then HIIT is an excellent choice. Just make sure that you weigh your priorities before making a decision.

Understand that the number of calories you burn in each cardio bout will be rather modest. A typical 180-pound (82 kg) male will expend about 350 calories over the course of a 45-minute cardio session. Although this certainly will help you control weight, it's not going to get you shredded. You can, of course, bump up caloric expenditure by upping the intensity or duration. Unfortunately, this also increases the risk of compromising muscle development. Only you can decide whether this tradeoff is worthwhile.

TIMING OF CARDIO

Another important consideration of concurrent training is when to perform the cardio component. You have two choices:

1. Schedule cardio on your days off from resistance training, or
2. include cardio on your lifting day.

Which is best? The short answer is that it really doesn't matter. Given the low-volume, low-intensity nature of the MAX cardio routine, both are viable options. Do whatever fits your lifestyle.

Performing cardio on days when you're not lifting has its benefits. It reduces the length of your training session. Shorter training sessions allow you more freedom to attend to non-gym matters on any given training day. This is particularly beneficial if you work long hours or have a hectic personal schedule. On the downside, however, you'll be exercising pretty much every day of the week, which, depending on your perspective, may not be an attractive alternative.

Prefer to perform cardio on your lifting day? No problem. Just follow one basic rule: always lift first. Even low-intensity cardio can sap vital energy reserves. You lose that extra oomph that you could otherwise draw on to push yourself, ultimately reducing the intensity of your lifts.

An even bigger concern may be that cardio drains glycogen reserves. The significance of this effect is that lifting weights in a glycogen-depleted state has been shown to decrease anabolic drive. AMPK seems to be responsible, at least in part, for this phenomenon. If you recall, AMPK interferes with pathways involved in muscle protein synthesis. What's a primary activator of AMPK? That's right—low levels of glycogen! The lower your glycogen levels, the more AMPK activity revs up.

The good news is that these effects become irrelevant as long as you perform the cardio following your weight workout. To maximize the anabolic response, consume your postworkout drink before the cardio bout. You can even sip on the drink as you perform the cardio. This will ensure that you take advantage of the anabolic window that exists after an intense resistance training session.

Another option is to split up the two components and perform cardio in the morning and resistance training later in the day (or vice versa). This is fine if you're able to accommodate such a schedule. After several hours of inactivity, your body has time to replenish its resources. Fatigue should not be an issue as long as your nutrition regimen is sound.

The Fasting Cardio Myth

A popular fat-loss strategy is to perform aerobic exercise first thing in the morning on an empty stomach. The rationale for the strategy is that a prolonged absence of food reduces circulating blood sugar, causing glycogen (stored carbohydrate) levels to fall. With less available glycogen, your body has no choice but to rely more on fat, rather than glucose, to fuel your workout. Moreover, the low insulin levels associated with fasting facilitate an environment that is favorable to fat breakdown, increasing the availability of fatty acids to be used as energy during the exercise session.

Unfortunately, what may seem like a sound strategy doesn't transfer into practice. Studies show that although a greater breakdown of fat takes place when you have fasted than after you have eaten, the rate of breakdown exceeds your body's ability to use the extra fatty acids for fuel. In other words, a lot of extra fatty acids that the working muscles can't use are floating around in the blood. Ultimately, these fatty acids are repackaged into triglycerides during the postworkout period and then shuttled back into fat cells. In the end you've gone to excessive lengths only to wind up at the same place you started.

More importantly, it's shortsighted to simply look at the number of fat calories you burn during an exercise session. Your metabolism doesn't operate in a vacuum. Rather, the body continually adjusts its use of fat and carbohydrate for fuel depending on a variety of factors. As a general rule, if you burn more carbohydrate during an exercise session, you'll ultimately burn a greater amount of fat in the postworkout period and vice versa. This begs the question, who cares if you burn a few extra fat calories while exercising if an hour later the ratio shifts to a greater carbohydrate utilization? In the end, it doesn't make a bit of difference. Bottom line: You need to evaluate fat burning over the course of days, not on an hour-to-hour basis, to get a meaningful perspective on its effect on body composition.

On top of everything, fasted cardio can have a catabolic effect on muscle. Studies show that training in a glycogen-depleted state substantially increases the amount of tissue proteins burned for energy during exercise (Blomstrand and Saltin 1999). Protein losses can exceed 10 percent of the total calories burned over the course of a one-hour cardio session—more than double that when training in the fed state. Any way you slice it, sacrificing your hard-earned muscle in a futile attempt to burn a few extra calories from fat doesn't make a whole lot of sense—especially if your goal is maximal muscle development!

CHOOSING A CARDIO MODALITY

Variety is an important element in all fitness activities, and cardiovascular exercise is no exception. With respect to cardio, variety is referred to as *cross-training*. Cross-training is best accomplished by alternating your workouts between two or more activities. Not only does this help stave off exercise boredom, it reduces wear and tear on your joints. Realize that aerobic activity is basically a repetitive-motion task, similar to continually typing on a keyboard (which, as we all know, can lead to carpal tunnel syndrome). Only by changing movement patterns can you spare your joints and connective tissue from continual impact and thus reduce the risk of injuries related to overuse.

You can use any continuous, submaximal activities for the MAX cardio component. Jogging, rowing, elliptical training, jumping rope, and many other modalities all make excellent choices. Remember that incorporating movements that involve both the upper and lower body helps maximize results.

Ideally, you should choose exercises that you enjoy. Enjoyment encourages adherence; the more you like an activity, the greater chance you'll keep doing it over time. That said, keep an open mind. Try out different activities; you may find that you enjoy an exercise more as time goes on.

References

Chapter 1

Petrella, J.K., Kim, J.S., Mayhew, D.L., Cross, J.M., & Bamman, M.M. (2008). Potent myofiber hypertrophy during resistance training in humans is associated with satellite cell-mediated myonuclear addition: A cluster analysis. *Journal of Applied Physiology,104*(6), 1736-1742.

Schoenfeld, B.J. (2010). The mechanisms of muscle hypertrophy and their application to resistance training. *Journal of Strength and Conditioning Research,24*(10), 2857-2872.

Sternlicht, E., Rugg, S., Fujii, L.L., Tomomitsu, K.F., & Seki, M.M. Electromyographic comparison of a stability ball crunch with a traditional crunch. *Journal of Strength and Conditioning Research, 21*(2) 506-509.

Willardson, J.M., Norton, L., & Wilson, G. (2010). Training to failure and beyond in mainstream resistance exercise programs. *Strength and Conditioning Journal, 32*(3) 21-29.

Chapter 2

Behm, D.G., Anderson, K., & Curnew, R.S. (2002). Muscle force and activation under stable and unstable conditions. *Journal of Strength and Conditioning Research,16*(3), 416-422.

Krieger, J.W. (2010). Single vs. multiple sets of resistance exercise for muscle hypertrophy: A meta-analysis. *Journal of Strength and Conditioning Research, 24*(4), 1150-1159.

Logan, P.A. & Abernethy, P.J. (1996). Timecourse changes in strength and indices of acute fatigue following heavy resistance exercise [Abstract]. *Australian Conference of Science and Medicine in Sport,* 28-31.

Chapter 8

Farinatti, P.T. & Castinheiras Neto, A.G. The effect of between-set rest intervals on the oxygen uptake during and after resistance exercise sessions performed with large- and small-muscle mass. *Journal of Strength and Conditioning Research, 25*(11) 31.

Chapter 9

Schoenfeld, B. (2011). The use of specialized training techniques to maximize muscle hypertrophy. *Strength and Conditioning Journal, 33*(4) 60.

Chapter 10

Campbell, B., Kreider, R.B., Ziegenfuss, T., La Bounty, .P, Roberts, M., Burke, D., Landis, J., Lopez, H., & Antonio, J. International Society of Sports Nutrition Position Stand: Protein and Exercise. *International Society of Sports Nutrition Position Stand: Protein and Exercise, 4*(8).

Churchley, E.G., Coffey, V.G., Pedersen, D.J., Shield, A., Carey, K.A., Cameron-Smith, D., & Hawley, J.A. (2007). Influence of preexercise muscle glycogen content on transcriptional activity of metabolic and myogenic genes in well-trained humans. *Journal of Applied Physiology,102*(4), 1604-1611.

Creer, A., Gallagher, P., Slivka, D., Jemiolo, B., Fink, W., & Trappe, S. Influence of muscle glycogen availability on ERK1/2 and Akt signaling after resistance exercise in human skeletal muscle. *Journal of Applied Physiology, 99*(3) 950–956.

Gorelick-Feldman, J., Maclean, D., Ilic, N., Poulev, A., Lila, M.A., Cheng, D., & Raskin, I. (2008). Phytoecdysteroids increase protein synthesis in skeletal muscle cells. *Journal of Agricultural and Food Chemistry,56*(10), 3532-3537.

Rivellese, A.A., De Natale, C., & Lilli, S. (2002). Type of dietary fat and insulin resistance. *Annals of the New York Academy of Sciences, 967,* 329-335.

Chapter 11

Blomstrand, E. & Saltin, B. Effect of muscle glycogen on glucose, lactate and amino acid metabolism during exercise and recovery in human subjects. *Journal of Physiology, 514* 293–302.

Heden, T., Lox, C., Rose, P., Reid, S., & Kirk, E.P. (2011). One-set resistance training elevates energy expenditure for 72 h similar to three sets. *European Journal of Applied Physiology, 111*(3), 477-484.

Kwon, H.R., Min, K.W., Ahn, H.J., Seok, H.G., Koo, B.K., Kim, H.C., & Han, K.A. (2010). Effects of aerobic exercise on abdominal fat, thigh muscle mass and muscle strength in type 2 diabetic subject. *Korean Diabetes Journal, 34*(1), 23-31.

Laye, M.J., Thyfault, J.P., Stump, C.S., & Booth, F.W. (2007). Inactivity induces increases in abdominal fat. *Journal of Applied Physiology, 102*(4), 1341-1347.

Trapp, E.G., Chisholm, D.J., Freund, J., & Boutcher, S.H. (2008). The effects of high-intensity intermittent exercise training on fat loss and fasting insulin levels of young women. *International Journal of Obesity (London), 32*(4), 684-691.

About the Author

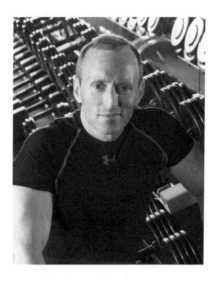

Brad Schoenfeld, MSc, CSCS, CPT, is widely regarded as one of the leading strength and fitness experts in the United States. The 2011 NSCA Personal Trainer of the Year is a lifetime drug-free body-builder who has won numerous natural bodybuilding titles, including the All-Natural Physique and Power Conference (ANPPC) Tri-State Naturals and USA Mixed Pairs crowns. As a trainer, he has worked with numerous elite-level physique athletes, including many top pros.

Schoenfeld is the author of eight other fitness books, including *Women's Home Workout Bible, Sculpting Her Body Perfect, 28-Day Body Shapeover,* and the best-seller *Look Great Naked* (Prentice Hall Press, 2001). He is a former columnist for *FitnessRX for Women* magazine, has been published or featured in virtually every major fitness magazine (including *Muscle and Fitness, MuscleMag, Ironman, Oxygen,* and *Shape*), and has appeared on hundreds of television shows and radio programs across the United States. He also serves as a fitness expert and contributor to www.bodybuilding.com, www.diet.com, and www.t-nation.com.

Certified as a strength and conditioning specialist by the National Strength and Conditioning Association and as a personal trainer by both the American Council on Exercise and the American College of Sports Medicine, Schoenfeld was awarded the distinction of master trainer by IDEA Health and Fitness Association. He is also a frequent lecturer on both the professional and consumer levels. He is currently pursuing his PhD in health science at Rocky Mountain University, where his research focuses on the mechanisms of muscle hypertrophy and their application to resistance training.

Visit his blog at www.workout911.com

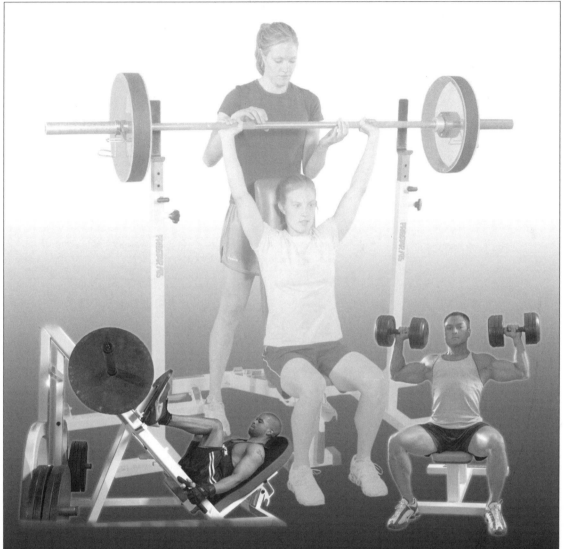

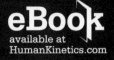